"Eons of accumulated feminine wisdom, having been muddled and dispersed by modern medical practice, have become sadly unavailable to today's woman. In this and in each of her books, Ms. Gaskin, one of the world's foremost scholars of such wisdom, puts it concisely and lovingly back into our hands. *Ina May's Guide to Breastfeeding* is the perfect gift for any pregnant woman. It is like having the best childbirth and lactation consultant right there at your bedside. And for nonpregnant women and men alike, may it be viewed as the seminal feminist text that it is, and may the reempowerment of women with respect to childbirth be seen as central to the work of feminism, and indeed the cause of humanity, in the twenty-first century."

—ANI DiFRANCO

"Ina May Gaskin is an international treasure. Her new guide to breastfeeding is the best thing ever written on the subject: a must-have for all pregnant women interested in the best start for their babies."

—CHRISTIANE NORTHRUP, M.D., author of
Women's Bodies, Women's Wisdom

ALSO BY INA MAY GASKIN

Ina May's Guide to Childbirth

Spiritual Midwifery

INA MAY'S
GUIDE TO
BREASTFEEDING

INA MAY'S
GUIDE TO
BREASTFEEDING

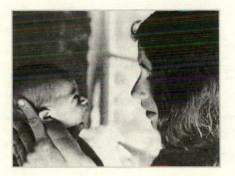

INA MAY GASKIN

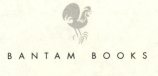

BANTAM BOOKS

NEW YORK

A Bantam Books Trade Paperback Original

Published in the United States by Bantam Books, an imprint of
The Random House Publishing Group, a division of Random House, Inc., New York.

BANTAM BOOKS and the rooster colophon are registered trademarks of Random House, Inc.

Image credits and permissions appear on pages 323 and 324.

Library of Congress Cataloging-in-Publication Data
Gaskin, Ina May.
Ina May's guide to breastfeeding / Ina May Gaskin.
p.   cm.
ISBN 978–0–553–38429–1
1. Breastfeeding. 2. Breastfeeding—Psychological aspects. 3. Attachment behavior.
I. Title. II. Title: Guide to breastfeeding.
RJ216.G275 2009
649'.33—dc22   2009017328

Printed in the United States of America

www.bantamdell.com

6   8   9   7   5

Book designed by Diane Hobbing

*To all those who work to raise the status of
breastfeeding as a gift for future generations*

CONTENTS

INA MAY'S
GUIDE TO
BREASTFEEDING

INTRODUCTION: BREAST IS BEST

Pregnancy can be a time of great wonder and excitement as you prepare for the birth of your baby. One of the great blessings of pregnancy is that your body and nature take complete care of the nourishment of your little one during his time inside your body (as long as you eat well). Who could design a machine that could reproduce and nourish its offspring so beautifully as this? You don't even have to think about how to do it!

One decision that *does* merit a conscious choice on your part is the first food that will nurture your baby once he is born. Will it continue to come from you or will you buy it from the shelves of a grocery store? Does it matter? You probably wouldn't have picked up this book if you didn't already have some idea of the benefits of breastfeeding and the possible undesirable consequences of feeding artificial milks to babies as a first choice. Even so, you may be surprised to find out how much your decision matters.

Assuming that pediatricians are the accepted medical experts on the needs and health of babies and young children, let's start with what their professional organization has to say on the subject of infant feeding. The American Academy of Pediatrics issued its first policy statement in support of breastfeeding in 1977, and in 1997 it followed up with a much stronger statement. In 2005 the AAP found it necessary to replace its 1997 policy statement with a newer version, because so many important recent studies corroborated what common sense had always recognized—that breast is best.[1]

Excerpts from the American Academy of Pediatrics' Policy Statement on Breastfeeding and the Use of Human Milk

- Human milk is the preferred feeding for all infants, including premature and sick newborns, with rare exceptions.

- When direct breastfeeding is not possible, expressed human milk, fortified when necessary for the premature infant, should be provided.

- Breastfeeding should begin as soon as possible after birth, usually within the first hour. Except under special circumstances, the newborn infant should remain with the mother throughout the recovery period. Procedures that may interfere with breastfeeding or traumatize the infant should be avoided or minimized.

- Newborns should be nursed whenever they show signs of hunger, such as increased alertness or activity, mouthing, or rooting. Crying is a late indicator of hunger.

- Appropriate initiation of breastfeeding is facilitated by continuous rooming-in.

- No supplements (water, glucose water, formula, and so forth) should be given to breastfeeding newborns unless a medical indication exists.

- Exclusive breastfeeding is ideal nutrition and sufficient to support optimal growth and development for approximately the first six months after birth.

Now let's turn to another health authority, the World Health Organization (WHO). The WHO ranks the safety of milks in the following way: first, the baby's mother's milk taken directly by the baby from the mother's breast; second, the baby's mother's milk taken from a bottle; third, the milk of another mother; and last, bottle-feeding of artificial milk formulas. Please note that the WHO does not say that artificial milk formulas shouldn't be consumed but that it is better for the baby if they are used only as a last resort.

Here is a very practical reason to begin nursing your baby. When you choose to feed your baby this way, you are preserving your ability to have a choice about your feeding method. *You can always stop breastfeeding and switch to artificial feeding later.* What is there to lose? On the other hand, if you begin with artificial feeding and then find that your baby is allergic to several different products (which happens sometimes), it can be quite difficult to switch back to breastfeeding.

Artificial Milks Don't Measure Up to Human Milk for Babies

It should not come as any surprise that the most desirable milk for a human baby is human milk. It is the most complete and perfect food for babies, just as camel milk is best for baby camels and cow's milk is best for calves. Breast milk even tastes better to young humans than other milks do. I've met many adults who were breastfed until the age of four or five who can recall the taste of their mother's milk, and each remembers it as incredibly delicious. Do you know anyone who buys infant formula because it is so delicious or who even has fond memories of it? I don't.

The composition of breast milk varies from mother to mother, and the composition of a given mother's milk varies according to her baby's needs. This means that if your baby is born prematurely, your milk will automatically adjust itself to contain the most advantageous mix of nutrients for him at his particular stage of development. No matter how many claims a manufacturer of a substitute milk formula makes about its similarities to breast milk, any substitute milk, no matter what brand, is quite different from human milk and is an inferior food source for human babies. As the AAP says, the superiority of human milk for human babies stands whether we are talking about the baby's growth, its development, or all other short- and long-term outcomes.

Immunologically speaking, mother's milk is medicine as well as food. It contains living cells, many of which will coat the mucous membranes of your baby's entire digestive system, protecting him against all kinds of bacteria and viruses. Artificial milk products do not contain any living cells, because anything that once lived in any formula concoction was long since killed during the production process. The protection offered by breast milk is important because, during birth, your baby leaves the sterile environment of your womb and sticks his head out into the highly contaminated environment outside. His system is not fully prepared for this shock, and he can use all the protection he can get.

Exclusive breastfeeding (meaning that a baby consumes nothing but his mother's milk) until the age of six months will continue to protect your growing baby's digestive tract, reducing the risk of allergy-causing foreign proteins entering his system. Such protection is especially important in families with a history of allergies, whether these allergies manifest as asthma, a specific food allergy, dermatitis, or allergy rhinitis (runny nose). Some babies started on artificial milk have to be switched from brand to brand several times during the early weeks of life because of their inability to tolerate these products. After the age of six months, babies begin to produce enough of their own antibodies to protect their intestinal walls against food antigens that may cause allergies.

Another strong reason for the ideal of exclusive breastfeeding for six months is that babies' digestive systems are just not sufficiently developed before that time to digest solid foods well. Incomplete digestion can cause intestinal pain, diarrhea, gas, inconsolable crying, and, in severe cases, damage to the baby's intestinal tract.

Babies who get artificial formulas instead of mother's milk miss out on these benefits and are more open to infection. Strong evidence shows that in all populations, in both wealthy and poor countries, these babies will have a higher incidence and severity of many serious diseases, including bacterial meningitis, bacterial infection of the blood, diarrhea, respiratory-tract infection, serious gastrointestinal infection, middle-ear infection, urinary-tract infection, and late-onset infection in premature babies.[2-13] And, according to one study, preemies who are fed artificial milk formulas have a higher incidence of the kind of blindness (retinopathy of prematurity) that has long been associated with premature birth.[14-15] Published research has shown that more than 1,000 childhood deaths per year in the United States could be prevented through breast-feeding and that for every 1,000 bottle-fed babies in the United States, seventy-seven hospital admissions are likely to result. Compare this with the five hospital admissions that can be expected for every 1,000 breast-fed babies.[16]

And there's more. Several studies have suggested increased rates of sudden infant death syndrome in the first year of life, as well as a higher incidence of diabetes mellitus; childhood cancers such as leukemia, Hodgkin's disease, and lymphoma; overweight and obesity; asthma and high cholesterol levels in older children and adults who were fed artificial milks compared with those who got their mothers' milk.[17–22]

Breastfed babies are not only healthier; there is some evidence demonstrating that they tend to be more intelligent. Several studies on the development of intelligence in babies have shown that the feeding of artificial milks was associated with lower performance.[23–25] A study involving about three hundred premature babies who were too small to suckle compared those given breast milk with those who received formula through a tube. When the two groups were IQ-tested at the age of eight years and the mothers' social and educational status were taken into account, the breastfed children scored significantly higher on the IQ tests than their formula-fed counterparts did.

Does this mean that a baby who is bottle-fed on formula will not be as intelligent as his breastfed sibling? I certainly wouldn't go that far, especially if the formula-fed baby receives high-quality loving attention while being fed. It's possible that the bottle-fed babies in some of these studies received less of their mothers' touch while feeding, since bottles can be propped on pillows, leaving the mother free to do something else while her baby feeds. Babies need more than milk to thrive—they need love expressed through touch. Skin is our most sensitive organ, and touch is the first language we speak. There is a lot of evidence from studies of other mammals about how important licking and touch are to the good health and even survival of their newly born young, and there's plenty more showing that human babies who are cuddled and given plenty of touch when young grow up to be more comfortable "in their own skins" than those who grow up deprived of touch. My opinion is that babies fed on artificial milks, particularly preemies and babies under the age of three to four months, need to be held as close to the breast as breastfed babies are, so they get the cuddling and loving touch they need and deserve. This is true as well if Dad is the one holding the bottle.

Breastfeeding is also the best analgesic for babies. Mothers who breastfeed their babies during painful procedures—for example, the heel poke to draw blood (sometimes called the PKU screening), which is generally given to babies within the first ten days of life—often find that their babies cry little if at all.[26–27] The analgesic effects also extend to times when a baby has his first cold or flu and, like the rest of us, feels miserable. Breastfeeding then becomes an especially valued comfort for both mother and baby.

Artificial Milks Are Frequently Recalled

The Food and Drug Administration (FDA) has been busy for decades issuing statements about "recalls" of artificial milk products that have been contaminated in various ways or that lack essential ingredients. See Appendix B for a list of FDA and firm recalls and warnings that took place in the United States during the first decade of the twenty-first century. Between 1982 and 1994, there were twenty-two significant recalls of various brands of artificial milks in the United States, with seven of these involving contamination or ingredients that were potentially life-threatening to babies. If you do need to use formula feeding at some point, be a smart shopper.

It's important to remember that when certain lots of formula are listed as "recalled" on the FDA website, many packages and cans from that lot have already been bought and fed to babies. How many mothers go to the FDA website to make sure that they're not feeding their babies a contaminated product? Not many, but if you feed your baby formula, this is the smart thing to do. Such recalls have been going on for decades, and it seems likely that they will continue, if past experience is any indication. Need I say it? Breast milk has never had to be recalled.

Health Advantages for Mothers Who Breastfeed

As many biologists have pointed out, Mother Nature is no fool. Her design for breastfeeding provides health benefits for mothers as well as babies. One of the most important benefits has to do with the role played by the natural hormone oxytocin. It is released from the mother's pituitary gland during labor, rising to higher levels as the baby is being pushed out of the vagina and peaking with the expulsion of the placenta. When the baby stimulates the breasts by nuzzling and licking the nipple or by breastfeeding, even more oxytocin is released in the mother. It causes uterine contractions (sometimes called "afterpains"), which hasten the process of the uterus returning to its prepregnant size. When such contact between mother and baby is facilitated, the advantage for the mother is a much-reduced chance of late postpartum hemorrhage; oxytocin is nature's way of preventing hemorrhage following birth.[28] Women whose babies are fed on artificial milks miss out on this antihemorrhagic benefit. They also miss out on the suppression of ovulation and menstruation that accompanies unrestricted breastfeeding. At six months postpartum, women who have not had a period, are not supplementing with artificial milk regularly, and are not going longer than four hours between daytime feedings or longer than six hours between night feedings have less than a two percent chance of becoming pregnant.[29-31]

Moms who breastfeed generally return to their prepregnancy weight more quickly than those who don't.[32] They get to eat an extra 500 to 600 calories a day and still lose weight (which is rather nice if you enjoy eating). And many studies show that if you are a working mother who decides to breastfeed, you are likely to miss fewer days of work, because your baby will be healthier.

Breastfeeding also has a positive long-term impact on women's health. Women who don't breastfeed have an increased risk of both breast cancer and ovarian cancer later on in life.[33-38] One of the most fascinating studies in this area involves women from fishing villages near Hong Kong who had the unusual habit of breastfeeding only with the right breast. This custom enabled researchers to compare the fate of the women's breasts. The researchers found a fourfold, highly significant increased risk of cancer in the unsuckled breast after menopause. We're talking about the prevention of diseases that are often fatal and that are always terribly expensive in terms of human suffering and cost of health care. Moms who don't breastfeed also have a higher incidence of osteoporosis and hip fractures when they are postmenopausal.[39-41]

Imagine that: The breastfeeding mother is multitasking every time she feeds her baby. As she nourishes her child, she loses weight at a safe rate, gains a pretty effective contraceptive treatment, and reduces her risk of two kinds of potentially deadly cancer and the brittle bones and subsequent fractures that can occur during the period after menopause.

The Impact of Artificial Feeding on Your Time and Budget

Are you living on a tight budget? If so, you can save a significant amount of money by nursing your baby—it costs nothing beyond the slight increase in your daily caloric needs. At most, it will set you back a few extra cents per day versus the cost of feeding substitute milks. We're talking about $1,800 to $2,600 per year per baby, just to buy the formula. Mothers enrolled in the Women, Infants, and Children (WIC) assistance program who are not breastfeeding are often surprised to find out that their monthly allotment of formula does not suffice and that they must pay for the rest of what they need each month at the going rate. Those who are most strapped for funds may start diluting the formula to make it last or begin introducing solid food before their baby's digestive system is prepared to deal with it.

Formula companies have been incredibly successful for more than half a century in convincing people, including most of the medical profession, that their product is almost as good as mother's milk (while implying that breastfeeding is something that only a few lucky women can manage). Guess who pays for this propaganda? Answer: not only each family with a substitute-milk-fed baby but the entire society, because of health-care costs, the missed benefits of breast milk, and the pollution factor (more on this later). It's not a stretch to say that the U.S. government has for decades subsidized a mammoth industry that directly competes with mother's milk as a major national resource.

Breast milk is always available and never requires sterilization or heating—a huge advantage for you. Have you thought about how much time and energy this can save? I remember one father-to-be who wondered how much trouble it was going to be for his wife to sterilize her nipples before each feeding! If you have anyone with similar worries in your family, I suggest that you tell them about nature's design—special oil glands create an antimicrobial environment around your nipples.

Better yet, breast milk is naturally organic. Almost all of the artificial milks for babies on the market are not organic, which means that they are likely to contain toxic chemicals, antibiotics, and bovine growth hormone if produced in the United States. It *is* possible to buy organic cows' milk or soy formulas, but, as you might expect, these are more expensive and harder to find. And even an organic product may contain ingredients (corn syrup is an example) that you may not want your newborn to eat because of its negative effects on babies' general health.

Environmental Impact

Artificial milks are incredibly wasteful when produced on a mass scale. The following information comes from the website of the World Alliance for Breastfeeding Action:

- Packaging of baby milks wastes resources such as tin, paper, and plastic. If every baby in the United States was bottle-fed, almost 86,000 tons of tin plate would be used each year in the required 550 million discarded tin cans. Another 1,230 tons of paper would be used if these tin cans had paper labels.

- Feeding bottles, teats (nipples), and related equipment require plastic, glass, rubber, and silicon. In 1987, 4.5-million feeding bottles were sold in Pakistan alone. The number per baby is even greater in industrialized countries (most babies in the United States have at least six bottles). Furthermore, Western hospitals and consumers are increasingly using "one-trip" disposable bottles and nipples.

- Waste materials from the production of baby milks are rarely recycled, so they increase our disposal problems. The two most common disposal methods, landfill and incineration, cause their own pollution.

- Baby milks are the end product of a number of industrial processes. The energy used to create the temperatures needed for these processes and the mechanical procedures used for production cause air pollution (acid rain and greenhouse gases) and also use natural resources in the form of fuel.

- The milk and packaging materials often travel considerable distances before processing, and, once ready for the market, baby milks have to be transported to the consumer. Many countries import baby milk from thousands of miles away, causing considerable unnecessary pollution. Ecuador, for example, imports baby milks from the United States, Ireland, Switzerland, and the Netherlands.

- Water, bottles, and nipples have to be sterilized before use. Water and the energy to boil it are normally easily available in the Northern Hemisphere, but this is no reason to waste them. The energy usually comes from polluting nuclear and conventional power stations. In the Southern Hemisphere, water and fuel are often precious resources. A three-month-old bottle-fed baby needs more than one quart (one liter) of water a day for mixing with formula, and each artificially fed baby needs at least an extra 1,500 pounds (73 kg) of firewood or its equivalent per year.

- Manufacturers use huge amounts of paper and other resources to promote their baby milks.

All that, and we still have to count the environmental costs of maintaining the cows to produce the milk. The tremendous amount of land and resources used by the dairy industry are a major contributor to the pollution of our environment.

Let's compare this with the environmental impact of breastfeeding:

- Breast milk produces no waste: It is produced in the right amounts for the baby's needs.

- Mothers need only the smallest amount of extra energy to produce milk, which is often taken from body fat (even malnourished mothers can produce enough quality breast milk to feed a baby).

- Breast milk needs no extra packaging.

- Breast milk is ready to use at the right temperature.

- Breast milk does not have to be shipped around the world. A mother has a ready supply wherever she goes.

- Most women do not menstruate when breastfeeding and therefore need fewer sanitary pads, tampons, or cloths. This reduces the need for fibers, bleaching, packaging, and disposal. If a baby is unrestrictedly breastfed for six months and breastfeeding continues into the second year, the average mother will not have a period until her baby is at least fourteen months old.

What other human activity would permit you to give your baby the best possible nurturing and health protection at the same time that you enhance your own long-term health, provide the most economical infant food possible, and protect the natural environment?

Times of Crisis

Many families these days take the trouble to pack an emergency kit in case of a tornado, flood, hurricane, earthquake, or other natural disaster. Breastfeeding mothers have an obvious advantage here, because the perfect food for their babies is with them at all times.

A couple of weeks after Hurricane Katrina devastated New Orleans and the Gulf Coast in 2005, another powerful hurricane, Rita, appeared to be heading for Houston, Texas. The mayor of the city ordered everyone to evacuate, and within hours, a million and a quarter Houstonians were in their cars, inching along a freeway that was not designed to accommodate anything like this volume of traffic. It wasn't long before tens of thousands of radiators were boiling over. According to the news reports, many families, having failed to anticipate the major traffic jam, had neglected to bring enough water or other drinks along with them. I think I would have preferred to be a breastfeeding mother that day rather than one who depended on manufactured milks.

In late November 2006, a California family became stranded in their car in the Oregon mountains during an unusual series of heavy snow- and rainstorms. They waited for more than a week to be rescued. Finally, James Kim, the father, built a fire for his wife, their four-year-old, and their seven-month-old baby, and began hiking out to find help. Sadly, Mr. Kim died of hypothermia before he could reach help, but his family was rescued alive. His wife had managed to sustain the two children by breastfeeding them. "The fact that Kati Kim was able to breastfeed both of her children for the amount of time that they were stranded most likely was lifesaving for them.... Breast milk not only provides the calories needed to sustain life, it also helps prevent dehydration," said Dr. Sheela Geraghty, assistant professor of pediatrics and medical director at the Center for Breastfeeding Medicine at Cincinnati Children's Hospital Medical Center.

Given all of the health benefits for babies and mothers that come with exclusive breastfeeding, you might wonder whether any countries have enacted national policies to make breastfeeding easier for mothers. The answer is yes. Norway, for instance, is a highly developed, wealthy country that has managed to successfully reclaim breastfeeding as the norm for babies. In 1970, only twenty percent of Norwegian babies were breastfed, a similar proportion to U.S. babies at the same time. Today, almost all Norwegian babies get their mothers' milk as their first food, and eighty percent of these babies are still being nursed by their mothers six months later. It is important to recognize that Norway accomplished this major change in its health policy without keeping mothers of young children confined to their homes or setting women with different viewpoints against one another. Much of that country's success can be attributed to wise public policies created by a coalition of physicians, feminists, and legislators, who all agreed that the lost art of breastfeeding ought to be revived for the good of babies and their mothers. See Chapter 15 for more information on how Norway learned to make breastfeeding easier for its mothers.

Closer to home is a Tennessee village called "The Farm," where I have lived and worked as a community midwife for several decades. Since the beginnings of my village, in 1971, virtually every woman there has breastfed her baby for at least the first several months. Of the first group of almost a thousand women, everyone nursed for at least a year, with only a handful of exceptions. At The Farm today, every woman expects to be able to breastfeed, because she knows literally hundreds of women who nursed their babies as long as they wished.

Were the women in my village a favored type of human to have had such success at breastfeeding when so many experience various difficulties in other parts of the United States? Actually, our breastfeeding mothers have always been an ordinary mix of young adults, as far as physical attributes go. What was unusual about us was that as a group, in the pioneering days of our community—when we were laying down the foundations and values of our lifestyle—we put ourselves into a situation that *required* every woman to breastfeed for the health and safety of her baby. During these early years, we had neither electricity nor running water, so it was virtually impossible to feed our babies with formulas. It turned out that the women in our group were able to reliably produce enough milk to fully nourish their babies—real-life evidence that breastfeeding works very well when conditions are right and small challenges are addressed before they become big problems. This allowed each new mother to begin nursing without the fear of failure.

My hope is that it is reassuring for you to know that a sizable group of women has had nearly one hundred percent success in breastfeeding in the modern world. This should let you know that there's nothing wrong with nature's design. Our experiences living as a community at The Farm provided us with some valuable insights about women's and babies' needs in the time after birth. What I consider most valuable about our circle of women's experience in recovering the female capacity to breastfeed is that it demonstrates what might be needed to reestablish a culture of breastfeeding in areas of the world where such a culture no long exists. I will bring up this community experience in later discussions throughout the book, because of the lessons that can be drawn from it for people living in entirely different circumstances.

Millions of people have been and still are negatively affected by the huge loss in breastfeeding in the United States during the first half of the twentieth century. My aim in this book is to inform you as well as possible in order to insulate you against the negative influences and senseless taboos that have become part of North American culture over the last few decades. At the same time, I hope to provide you with practical information about how breastfeeding works, making it easier and more enjoyable for you and your baby.

A Note About Gender

In alternate chapters, I will switch between using feminine or masculine pronouns when referring to your baby.

A Note About Etiquette

Although I strongly advocate that new parents make every effort to nurse their babies, as a matter of compassion I also believe it's important for those of us who breastfeed to refrain from being judgmental of those who do not. How would it make you feel for someone to make comments about a way of feeding that you have no way to reverse? It is possible to educate without issuing statements that make people feel criticized.

1

How Breastfeeding Works,
and How It Relates to Mothering

We women are all born with the right equipment for breastfeeding. Big breasts, tiny breasts, long nipples, flat nipples, light nipples, and dark nipples all work very well for milk-making and breastfeeding. The basic milk-producing equipment is present in all the variations that we see in the human female. Why, then, is it so much easier for some women to breastfeed than it is for others? This chapter is intended to give you a foundation for understanding why this is so. There are external factors that can interfere with your innate ability to nurse your baby, but the important thing for you to remember is that these have nothing to do with the body you are dealt at birth, which has the capacity to work right.

Breasts are amazing, complex organs, which are able to produce, secrete, and deliver the most perfect food possible to your baby, who is hardwired to take it in. Your breasts are even talented enough to adjust the composition of your milk according to the gestational age of your baby at birth and to the amount of heat and humidity in your environment at any given moment.

Let's take a quick look now at the different kinds of tissues that make up your breasts. First there is the glandular tissue of your breasts, the network of grapelike clusters (alveoli) and ducts that make the milk and move it along. Next, your breasts contain a web of ligaments that help to support their weight. Then there are the nerves of the breast and nipple, which make them sensitive to touch. It is this network of nerves that responds to your baby's nuzzling, suckling, head-bobbing, and caressing, by sending the message to your pituitary gland to secrete prolactin, the hormone that signals your breasts to make milk. You'll probably learn later on that your baby's cry and even the thought of your baby can do the same thing. The rest of your breast tissues are the more-liquid components: the blood, which nourishes all the rest of the tissues and provides the nutrients needed to make milk, and the lymph, which removes wastes.

By the way, none of the tissues mentioned so far has anything to do with the size of your breasts. Breast size depends upon the amount of fatty tissue in your breasts, not upon the amount of glandular (milk-making) tissue. Some of us have a lot of fat in our breasts, while others have more-moderate amounts or very little. The amount of fat has no effect on our ability to make milk. Pregnancy means dramatic breast growth in some women, but women who still have tiny breasts at the end of pregnancy are quite able to fully breastfeed their babies.

Your nipple sticks out from your areola; it is in the middle of the darker-colored part of your breast. Both nipple and areola contain erectile muscle tissue. When your nipple is stimulated by touch, cold, or a visual or auditory cue, these muscles contract, and your nipple becomes hard and erect. Once your baby takes it into her mouth properly, it will take on an entirely different shape, doubling in length and conforming to the shape of your baby's mouth cavity.

Hormones That Affect Lactation and How to Elicit Them

It takes more than the right "equipment" to make milk—it is also necessary for that equipment to get the signal that it is time to start producing and releasing the milk. This is the job of certain hormones that are produced in the body, hormones that may rise or fall according to the mother's stress level and the atmosphere in which she first starts suckling her baby.

Oxytocin

The hormone oxytocin plays as large a role in lactation and mothering as it does in the process of labor and birth. When you feel your uterus contract during or after labor, you are feeling just one of the many effects of oxytocin: in this case, the ability to expel something from a bodily organ. Oxytocin not only stimulates the muscles of the uterus to expel the baby at the culmination of labor, it also stimulates the muscles of the breast to expel milk during nursing in what is called the "letdown reflex."

Oxytocin has been called the "hormone of calm, love, and healing" because of the kinds of feelings it causes in the mother and the interactions with her baby that often trigger its release.[1] For instance, it has been found that a newborn baby can cause additional oxytocin release

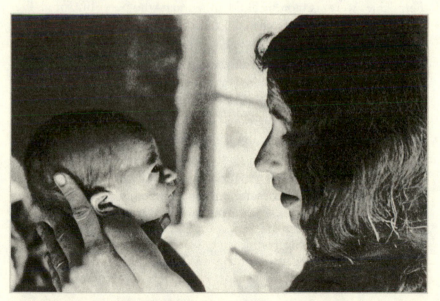

Mom and baby under the influence of oxytocin

in the mother's bloodstream by massaging, nuzzling, or licking her nipple. Both skin-to-skin contact and eye-to-eye communication between mother and baby also trigger the release of oxytocin. Under the influence of high oxytocin levels, mother and baby tend to stare at each other lovingly, provided that skin-to-skin contact—or only light clothing between them—is the norm just after birth and there are no distractions or interruptions.

Extremely high levels of oxytocin persist in the bloodstreams of mother and baby for about an hour after vaginal birth, giving both a feeling of well-being and gratitude. Higher levels than usual will persist throughout the nursing period, as long as the mother doesn't have extremely high levels of stress (since high levels of stress hormones inhibit the secretion of oxytocin).

And though severe stress can sometimes inhibit the release of oxytocin, research has also shown that oxytocin often *lowers* stress in lactating women by slowing the heart rate and reducing blood pressure. There is evidence that the powerful calming effect that breastfeeding can have on a mother during the early weeks of life is long-lasting: Dr. Kerstin Uvnäs Moberg, a Swedish oxytocin researcher, found that women who breastfed their babies for the first seven weeks were calmer when their babies were six months old than women who never breastfed. Her research team also found that small amounts of oxytocin reduce anxiety and increase curiosity and a willingness to relate with another being. In Moberg's words, "Oxytocin is physiology's 'forget-me-not' that makes recognition and bonding reverberate in the nerves' pathways." Larger amounts of oxytocin, such as that which a mother and baby might experience during a longer nursing session, produce a more pronounced calming effect—a tendency to move around less, to relax and rest. The same research team discovered that oxytocin also alleviates pain. When a rat is given repeated oxytocin injections, it will take longer than usual to pull its tail out of water that is too hot. Oxytocin's ability to reduce pain applies to both mother and baby and is a blessing that is quite noticeable when a breastfed baby must undergo a painful medical test or a new mother is healing after a cesarean.[2]

Are you surprised that one hormone can do so many different things related to nurturing and parenting? Actually, it can do all that and more. To illustrate what I mean, it is worth knowing that we women have the ability to produce oxytocin even when we aren't pregnant. (Men can produce it, too, but its effects are more pronounced in females.) Oxytocin levels in the body rise when we enjoy a good meal (when we take the time to focus on it), whether alone or in the company of people we enjoy. It is no accident that business people consummate so many deals around a shared meal, as eating together causes oxytocin levels to rise, thus instilling a sense of calm and trust that makes it easier for people to cooperate with one another.

Another stimulus to oxytocin release in both sexes is pleasant, rhythmic touch. Much research has confirmed that oxytocin levels rise when we receive a hug from someone we care for or a soothing massage, as well as during meditation, a warm bath, or sexual arousal. As oxytocin levels rise, blood pressure drops, heart rate slows, and the digestive system functions at maximum efficiency. The same goes for healing: Our bodies heal better when oxytocin levels are high and our stress hormones are at a low ebb. When we are under the influence of oxytocin, problems that may have been bothering us previously tend to move into the background, and we may view our situation in a more positive way. We may also feel an enhanced sense of closeness to others and an impulse to greater generosity.

Consider the experience of Jiang Xiaojuan, the twenty-nine-year-old Chinese policewoman who was called a national hero by the media after the Jiangyou earthquake of May 2008. Officer Xiaojuan nursed nine babies whose mothers were injured or killed in the earthquake. For Officer Xiaojuan, whose own son was six months old, it was a simple matter. "I am breastfeeding," she said, "so I can feed babies. I didn't think of it much. It is a mother's reaction and a basic duty as a police officer to help."

While she was bemused about the media fuss over her actions, she did allow that she felt something special for these little ones: "I feel about these kids I fed just like my own. I have a special feeling for them. They are babies in a disaster." I'm sure that this policewoman's actions were prompted not only by a sense of duty but also by the increased level of oxytocin that she experienced when she encountered the hungry babies. Her milk flowed in greater quantities than usual because she felt a need to feed these helpless little ones.

All mammals share the ability to produce oxytocin, and expressions of maternal kindness and generosity are not limited to our own species. The Sriracha Zoo near Bangkok, Thailand, has attracted a lot of media

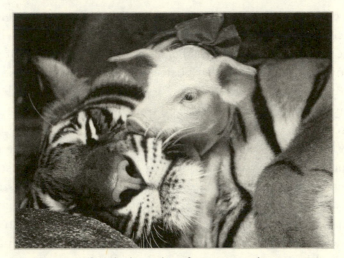

Oxytocin-induced relationship of nurturing and trust

attention in recent years for its cross-species suckling arrangements. Zookeepers there apparently do a certain amount of intentional "baby-snatching," which is then followed by successful foster relationships that zoo visitors find entertaining. From this, we get the improbable sight of a sow suckling tiger cubs or of a six-year-old royal bengal tigress (who was suckled by a pig for her first four months of life) suckling six piglets and behaving as any loving, protective mother would toward her charges. Clearly, the zookeepers rely on the power of oxytocin to pull off such stunts.

Who wouldn't want to have high oxytocin levels during pregnancy and birth? This is best accomplished by having as much contact with your baby as possible right after birth. As mentioned, skin-to-skin contact is best, but even with clothes on and your baby wrapped in a receiving blanket, your oxytocin levels can be enhanced by just holding and caressing her. If you have had a stressful birth, holding and cuddling your baby will usually improve the way you feel almost instantly. One of the few exceptions to this would be if you feel so weak following birth that you are on the point of fainting. Common sense, of course, should rule in these matters. The amount of contact you have with your baby just after birth may vary according to whether you gave birth vaginally and whether your perineum needs stitching. However, women who have cesareans or need perineal repair will also benefit by both seeing and touching their babies as much as possible in the moments soon after birth.

More generally, the way to have a high level of oxytocin after birth is to avoid stress. Here I'm not referring to the work or even the pain of birth. Rather, this means any factor—including the people assisting your birth—that interferes with your ability to connect with your baby once her breathing is spontaneous and unassisted. This is especially important during your child's first hour of life—a period of extraordinary sensitivity for both you and your baby, when your respective systems are meant to be in attunement.

Beta-endorphin

Beta-endorphin is another hormone that has an important function around the time of birth and breastfeeding. From ancient times, humans have known about opiates (drugs derived from the opium poppy) and their ability to kill pain and produce ecstatic states of consciousness. However, it wasn't until the mid-1970s that researchers discovered that the human body produces its own opiate: beta-endorphin. It is secreted by the pituitary gland and the hypothalamus in circumstances of stress, muscular effort, excitement, orgasm, and pain. Its properties are similar to those of morphine, heroin, and meperidine (Demerol), a painkiller commonly used in maternity wards in the United States, and it works on the same receptors of the brain. Anyone who follows sports closely is aware of the phenomenon that occurs when an athlete is injured on the playing field but is able to continue playing without feeling much pain. High levels of beta-endorphin are very effective at blocking pain receptors.

Beta-endorphin has another function: It facilitates the release of the hormone prolactin during labor, which prepares the mother's body for lactation and helps the baby's lungs finish their maturation process. Beta-endorphin is present in high levels for about three days following birth and then returns to its former level. However, it remains present in breast milk, which helps to account for the blissful expression we see on the faces of babies who have just enjoyed a good session at the breast.

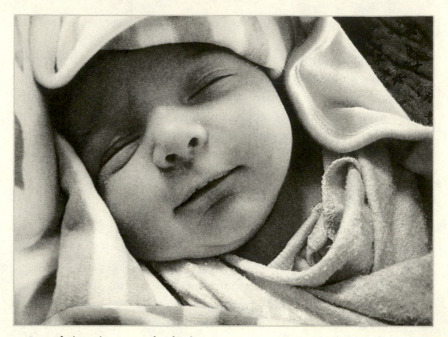

Breastfed newborn just after feeding

Prolactin

Now we come to prolactin, which has been called the "mothering" or "nesting" hormone. *Pro lactin,* incidentally, means *for milk* in Latin. It is released by the pituitary gland during pregnancy and lactation and prepares the pregnant woman's breasts for lactation by causing the maturation and proliferation of the mammary ducts and alveoli. High levels of the hormone progesterone inhibit the production of milk during pregnancy (though, in many women, not to the point of suppressing lactation if they are still nursing an older child). Progesterone and estrogen levels drop abruptly after birth, and prolactin causes the milk-producing cells in the mother's breasts to begin producing first colostrum and then milk.

Prolactin is related to other forms of mothering behavior as well. It has to do with nest building, grooming, and comforting. Michel Odent has written that while oxytocin creates a need to love, prolactin creates a tendency "to direct the effects of the love hormone toward babies."[3] Prolactin is likely to be the hormone that urges the mother to put her baby's needs first and foremost.

Other effects of prolactin include stimulating the secretion of oxytocin and natural painkillers such as beta-endorphin, and the suppression of fertility. Like oxytocin, prolactin also helps reduce stress—for both mother and baby.

Interestingly, men and women have similar prolactin levels when there is no pregnancy.[4] Studies have shown that fathers-to-be have increased prolactin levels, paralleling the increased levels of their partners. Holding babies appears to raise prolactin levels in men as well as women, and new fathers' prolactin levels also increase when they hear their babies' cries.[5-6] New fathers with high prolactin levels tend to be more responsive to their newborns' cries.

To sum up this discussion about the hormones that facilitate lactation, ease of breastfeeding is directly related to having high levels of oxytocin, beta-endorphin, and prolactin in the bloodstream around the time of birth. Nature endows each woman with the equipment to produce these hormones, but in stressful environments it can become more difficult for her to secrete them in the necessary amounts. This will be discussed later on in the chapter.

Colostrum

Baby's first drink, colostrum, is the thick yellowish milk that your breasts begin to produce—usually, but not always, in small amounts—during the last half of your pregnancy and for the first two or three days after birth. Colostrum is protein-packed. It gives way to what usually seems like more than enough milk in a day or two (sometimes three or four) after giving birth.

Do not worry about whether you can produce colostrum. Barring some sort of serious injury or radical surgery, it would be impossible for you not to.

Colostrum is full of antibodies, immune factors, enzymes, and other goodies that help to get your baby started well in life outside your body. Partly a laxative, it helps your baby expel the dark meconium, which is your baby's first poop. This action gets your baby's digestive system ready to receive the greater quantities of milk that will soon begin to fill your breasts.

Exclusive suckling from the mother (that is, no supplemental feeds or drinks of other kinds) works best for human babies. Most exclusively breastfed babies who have unlimited access to their mother's breast will drink only about an ounce during the first twenty-four hours after being born. That's about two tablespoons, or one-eighth of a cup. If you are not used to U.S. cooking measurements, the amount is less than what would fill an egg cup.

Colostrum's function is, in a way, more medicinal than nutritive. It is so important to newborn babies that even the mother who plans to bottle-feed her baby on an artificial milk would be well advised to give her baby only the colostrum from her breast for at least the first three days of life. Dr. Ruth Lawrence's research has shown significant correlations between increased asthma, urinary-tract and respiratory infections, gastrointestinal disease, later obesity, and juvenile-onset insulin-dependent diabetes when artificial formula is given to babies soon after birth.[7] When your baby swallows several mouthfuls of colostrum while nursing during the first two days, this small amount will maintain her blood sugar at the ideal level. It's good to remember that your newborn baby is still making the transition from being fed by the placenta to actively feeding at your breast, at the same time that your body is making the transition from pregnancy (storing food in your baby's vital organs) to lactation (producing food for your baby).

My friend who grew up on a farm, where her family raised sheep, told me that sometimes a ewe would give birth to the first of twins, and the firstborn would be too weak to get to its feet to reach its mother's teat. My friend learned to milk a small amount of colostrum into her palm and drip it into the weak lamb's mouth. Almost immediately, she said, the lamb would begin to suck on her fingers, and dull eyes became bright and weak legs strengthened—more evidence of the powerful effect that comes from even the tiniest amount of colostrum.

Sonja's story shows how colostrum also has immediate benefits for sick human babies:

Sonja: *When I learned I was pregnant, I already knew I wanted to have a natural birth. I couldn't wait to have a beautiful birth experience that would give my baby the best start into this world. When I ended up* with an emergency C-section, I had the most difficult time in my life instead. My baby boy was taken to the neonatal intensive care unit (NICU), and it was a long ten hours after his birth before I could even hold him in my arms for the first time.

I felt completely down when Eleanor, the breastfeeding consultant working for the hospital, entered my room and started talking to me about breastfeeding. She also showed me how to use the breast pump that was available in every room to stimulate milk production. Her words, her voice, and her calm energy were exactly what I needed to bring my focus back to being a mom for my baby. After my little baby boy latched on to my breast with ease, I gained a new powerful sense of motherhood. I still had something that only I could give to my precious boy—something that would help make him grow and get stronger.

I remember how later on, while I was breastfeeding my baby in the NICU, Eleanor went into my room to get the leftovers of my colostrum from the collection bottles. What I thought was just a few drops (not worth saving) amounted to a whole syringe full of colostrum. She brought it down to the neonatal care unit to store it in the refrigerator, explaining to the nurses the importance of breast milk, especially for the babies treated there. She said every drop was precious and mentioned that colostrum may even be used as a lotion for a baby's dry skin. As a result, I asked the nurses to call me every time my boy needed a shot or a new IV, so I could breastfeed him before each procedure. This greatly eased his discomfort—to the point that he sometimes ignored the pain completely and did not cry at all.

Thanks to Eleanor, I had enough strength to be there for my little boy during those long seven days in NICU. And now I cherish each moment I can hold my son in my arms while I feed him, calm him, and comfort him. The connection I feel when I nurse him helps me forget the difficult past and gives me a feeling I would not trade for anything in the world.

The Beginning of Milk Production

On day two or three after most births, your milk will come in. You'll know when this happens by the following signs: Your breasts will become warm and firm to the touch, and they will swell. Your baby, who suckled quietly when there was only colostrum in your breasts, may have to gulp at a fast rhythm to keep up with the flow. She will begin to pee larger amounts, and her poop will begin to change from the sticky dark meconium that clings to her skin to something that looks more like yellowish cottage cheese curds in yellow liquid. Breastfed-baby poop, unlike meconium, smells, but it's not really stinky.

Your milk may come in either sooner or later than expected without there being an abnormality. For example, milk usually comes in earlier in women who have breastfed a previous baby, and it often comes in a day or so later when birth takes place in a hospital (especially when the mother has had little close contact with her baby or has been able to suckle her baby only according to scheduled times rather than by the baby's cues).

Most women have the capacity to produce considerably more milk than one baby needs. Milk supply is directly related to the amount of milk that is removed and the frequency with which this happens—demand regulates supply. Your breasts don't know whether they will need to produce for one, two, or three babies, and, as with certain other mammals, nature has provided you with the capacity to feed two babies simultaneously. It may also reassure you to know that research has shown that even women who are themselves malnourished are able to produce a sufficient supply of good-quality milk for their babies. They need only drink to satisfy thirst in order to produce enough milk. The rest of the job is about releasing that milk.

To keep producing milk, though—once your breasts really go into full production and your baby's appetite is fully aroused—your breasts must receive the message of stimulation and, equally important, the removal of milk by suckling, manual expression, or pumping. If there is no frequent stimulation and removal, your milk will dry up over a few days.

The Letdown Reflex

When your baby suckles at your breast, the level of prolactin in your blood rises and stays high for the better part of an hour. This additional prolactin triggers the appropriate cells in your breast to make milk. Then comes a surge of oxytocin, which causes the contraction of the bandlike cells that surround the milk-making glandular tissue in your breast, squeezing the newly made milk into the duct system and out of your body. First-time mothers—like Franki, whose story is below—may be surprised and delighted to find out that they can shoot their milk several feet.

❧ **Franki:** *My first baby was three weeks old. I left for less than two hours to run some errands by myself, leaving the baby safe at home with Daddy. There I was in the grocery line, waiting to check out, fully armed with clothes, a good nursing bra, and breast pads, because my milk supply was bountiful from the time it came in. A lady and child behind me were arguing over gum, and the kid started crying and wailing, as some of them do at a time like that. Hearing that cry started my milk flowing, and by the time I got to the cashier, I was completely wet all the way through. My letdown was so strong I was actually tossing spots of milk on the floor and grocery conveyor belt as I unloaded my cart. The only thing that saved me from total embarrassment was that I knew the cashier, and we just laughed and laughed.*

Some women feel the letdown reflex, while others don't. Those who do feel it often describe it as a pleasurable sensation of warm tingling that moves from the breast cells close to the chest outward toward the nipple. But, as I implied above, it is possible for the milk-ejection reflex to be functioning perfectly without your feeling that tingle. (Smaller breasts tend to be more sensitive to this sensation than larger breasts.) Any baby who is well latched to the breast, sucking, and gulping is giving signals of a well-functioning milk-ejection reflex. You may have several letdowns in one feeding if your baby is sucking quite well. Multiple letdowns (whether you feel them or not) ensure that your baby gets the higher-protein, higher-fat hindmilk, which is let down after the thinner, more thirst-quenching foremilk.

Research has shown that the highest prolactin levels correlate with the times of higher milk production and that these occur between two A.M. and six A.M. after an evening of frequent breastfeeding with full emptying of both breasts.[8] For this reason, women wishing to increase milk production are advised to get in a feeding or pumping session during this time period. See page 108 for more information on the letdown reflex.

Breastfeeding, like Birth, Works Best
When Stress Levels Are Low

When I was nine, I spent an entire summer with my grandmother and Aunt Myra on an Iowa farm. In those days on family farms, milk cows had pleasant lives, spending their days in pastures rather than in cramped feed lots. One of my chores was to round up the cows in one of the outlying pastures at sundown and herd them back to the barn. My aunt, knowing how impatient nine-year-olds can be, put me under strict orders never to hurry the cows from the pasture into the barn. "Horses and ponies trot, and that's fine," she told me, "but if you try to make a milk cow move faster than she wants to go, she won't be able to let her milk down when she gets to the barn." Years later, I reflected on these instructions when I was suckling my own children and understood that I had internalized something important from them that helped me when I was in the early years of my midwifery work. Milk flows best and most abundantly when the mother's needs are understood and respected.

Several stress factors that are common to modern life can interfere with a woman's ability to breastfeed. More often than not, these can be overcome, but it is necessary for you to know what they are so you can do everything possible to avoid piling up too many of them.

Stress Hormones

Every species of mammal needs the stress hormones that our bodies produce—adrenaline and cortisol—to help respond to dangerous situations, just as much as we need oxytocin and prolactin to help calm ourselves, recover from being in stress mode too long, and nurture our young. The calming and the stress hormonal systems are both part of the innate makeup of both genders, and ideally they should balance each other out. Adrenaline and cortisol cause several responses to occur simultaneously: Blood pressure rises, the heart beats faster, digestion slows down, and the organism becomes mentally alert and ready to fight or flee instantaneously.

Breastfeeding is easiest when the mother is not stressed—when, in fact, her family and the rest of her society give her encouragement and friendly support. If a mother is full of stress hormones, her oxytocin and prolactin levels will be greatly inhibited and her milk production may be much reduced or even temporarily stopped, as Melissa's story shows.

Melissa: *Baby Jeffrey was weighed and measured at his first well-child checkup at five days old. He nursed during the appointment, and milk was dripping from both of my breasts. Everything was fine, as we had expected, until the end of the checkup, when the doctor pulled out a weight chart and began to tap the buttons on his calculator watch. He said that Jeffrey had lost nearly ten percent of his body weight. He asked again if I was breastfeeding, and I told him that I was. Then the doctor told me that I should give Jeffrey a bottle in addition to nursing until his weight came up. I said that I didn't want to do that—I wanted to breastfeed.*

"I know you want to breastfeed," he said. "Those Birkenstocks show me that you're a hippie. But if you want to keep trying, you'll have to go to the lactation consultant to make sure that it is all right." Off we went to the hospital.

The lactation consultant weighed Jeffrey before and after I nursed him. She said that he was getting only a tiny bit of milk. Not enough. She told me to feed him formula and went to her supply closet, which was full of formula, and got some. I sat in the chair and cried. She didn't even look at me. I was sent home with formula and a tube, as I had still refused to accept a bottle for my five-day-old son.

My milk dried up that afternoon from the stress and fright of that morning. All night Jeffrey tried to nurse, and nothing came out for him. The next morning, exhausted and sad, we went back to the lactation consultant for our follow-up. There we fed Jeffrey with the lactation aid. At home later, I lay on the bed and fed him with the tube. I hated it.

That evening, after a full day without my milk, I got myself together and decided how to heal. My husband, baby, and I loaded up in the car and took a drive. We got a pizza and a movie—our usual routine for Friday. It felt really normal, and we relaxed. Late that night, my milk came back in. Jeffrey regained his birth weight by the time he was two weeks old.

I don't want you to think that all or even most lactation consultants or pediatricians would exhibit such uninformed attitudes toward breastfeeding. Many pediatricians and most lactation consultants would be aware that five-day-old babies usually haven't yet recovered their birth weight and that a mother whose breasts are dripping with milk should not be discouraged from breastfeeding. And most lactation consultants would also be able to distinguish between a baby who is doing well with breastfeeding and one who actually needs supplemental feedings. Newborn babies tend to lose a few ounces (five to seven percent of the baby's birth weight is average) during the first few days following birth, regardless of whether they are nursed or formula-fed. This weight loss is generally recovered by day ten to fourteen of life (if recovery of the lost weight takes more than two weeks, it's best to contact a lactation consultant).

There's a big difference between a baby who is a few days old and hasn't yet regained her birth weight and one who is two or three weeks old and still under her birth weight. What Melissa's story illustrates well is that her milk production and her milk-ejection reflex were both inhibited by the emotional upset caused by the lack of breastfeeding knowledge exhibited by this particular pediatrician and lactation consultant. The quick recovery of her milk supply when she decided not to be victimized by their words and advice was also a function of her return to a normal hormonal balance for a lactating mother.

I am certain that one of the reasons all the women in my community were able to breastfeed their babies was that we created a largely stress-free culture for women and babies without making life unpleasant for everyone else. To begin with, we didn't have to encounter negativity about breastfeeding within our community, because if anyone disapproved, nothing was said aloud. Nobody gave us nasty looks when they noticed that we were breastfeeding. There were no worried grandparents among us who were trying to change our minds about the wisdom of breastfeeding instead of feeding our babies with manufactured milks. Everyone in our community, including those who had no children or were newcomers, soon came to understand what mothers and nursing babies needed. If those who joined the community had hang-ups about breastfeeding, they soon got over them. We actually learned how to get the right mix of hormones before we ever knew what the names of the hormones were!

2

PREPARING FOR NURSING

Once you've made the decision to nurse your baby, what can you do during pregnancy to prepare for nursing? As discussed in the previous chapter, your body is doing most of the work for you, but there are some things that you can do to ease the transition.

You may be able to find a breastfeeding class in your area. If so, I would encourage you to find the time to take it if at all possible. Attending such a class is a good way to meet other pregnant women who are interested in nursing, and it will also give you the chance to watch some of the great nursing videos that are available today. An additional benefit is that in many of these classes you will have a chance to meet women who are successfully nursing. Women who have already breast-fed are a great source for practical information.

If you are the first person in your family to choose nursing, you may find that your decision meets with some resistance from family members. They may believe that you won't be able to produce enough milk or that you will be "hogging" the baby, or they may simply be uncomfortable about nursing because they have never or rarely seen it. If this is the case, the statistics in the introduction and the list of resources at the back of this book should be helpful in reassuring your worried relatives.

Breast Care During Pregnancy

Your breasts do a good job of taking care of themselves during pregnancy. In almost every case, the best thing to do is to leave well enough alone. Avoid washing your nipples with any kind of soap that might remove their natural lubrication. Your nipples actually need this lubrication, which is produced by the little oil glands on the areola that grow larger during pregnancy. These little glands—unique to the nipple—also help to maintain an acid balance, which is what creates the antimicrobial atmosphere of your nipples. Sometimes, well-meaning people advise women who intend to nurse to apply different ointments or substances, such as witch hazel or tincture of benzoin, that are supposed to toughen skin. This is a bad idea when it comes to nipple care, as these substances can dry the skin and cause it to crack. It is also a bad idea to rub your nipples hard with a towel to toughen them. Being this rough with them can actually remove the protective layers of skin that develop during pregnancy. If, for any reason, your nipples are *already* dry and in need of lubrication, you can apply some pure lanolin, but be careful not to cover the tip of your nipple.

One thing you can do to care for your breasts is to keep your nipples as dry as possible, particularly if you experience some leakage of colostrum. This will not be a problem for most women—though most will be able to express colostrum, it is comparatively rare for it to flow without being manually expressed. Generally, the only women who will experience the leakage of colostrum during pregnancy are those with large breasts, where the nipples are the lowermost part. If your breasts are like this, I suggest that you look for a bra that provides good support during pregnancy to minimize such leaking. Avoid wearing a bra with a plastic liner though, as this may irritate your breasts and keep your nipples from staying dry.

Whether you experience noticeable leakage of colostrum or not, a few drops of colostrum are likely to accumulate on the end of your nipple and dry there. This is a little like the dried goop that accumulates in the corner of your eyes during the night. You can remove it without scraping your nipple.

It's a good idea, when you are 34 to 36 weeks pregnant, to express several teaspoons of colostrum into a sterilized container and freeze it. If you should give birth before 39 to 40 weeks, this stored colostrum can help keep your premature or late-preterm baby from developing jaundice. Follow this same procedure if you are diabetic, as your baby will have an increased need for your colostrum, but start collecting and storing as early as 32 weeks. Such stimulation of the breast does not cause early labor.

If your nipples are quite sensitive beyond the first trimester of pregnancy, I suggest that you spend at least part of your day with them exposed to the air (and, if possible, to a little sunlight). If you are able to go bra-less during part of the day, the slight friction of your nipples against your clothes is a good kind of "nipple conditioning." In general, you should avoid tight, restrictive clothes, as they will irritate your sensitive nipples. Going bra-less during the night is also a good idea, as your lymphatic system functions best when there is no external pressure on the soft tissue of your torso. Take a towel to bed with you if there is leakage during the night.

Breast massage and stimulation of the breasts or nipples during sexual activity can also be a helpful preparation for nursing. If this is part of your normal lovemaking, there is no reason to discontinue it. Grasping of your nipples can build a protective layer of skin there, making them slightly less sensitive to touch. On the other hand, if you have a history of giving birth prematurely, it's good not to do any breast stimulation until your baby is no longer premature.

Checking Your Nipples

Are you afraid that the shape of your nipples will keep you from nursing? Here are a few techniques that will help you determine if you have flat, inverted, or retracted nipples. It's unlikely that any of these conditions will prevent you from nursing, but it's better for you to find out before your baby is born, since there are ways to reshape your nipples if they are severely inverted or retracted.

Here is a quick way to tell if your nipples are inverted or retracted. Grasp your nipple at the base between your thumb and forefinger and press your thumb and forefinger together several times. A flat nipple will remain flat when you do this. An inverted nipple will retreat farther

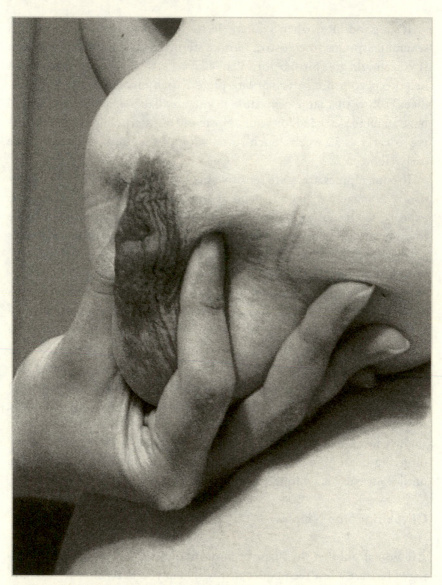

Pinching alone can't make this nipple erect.

inward. Another way you can tell is that flat and inverted nipples do not become erect when they are stimulated or cold.

If one or both of your nipples are flat, it is generally not necessary to take any action during pregnancy to correct this condition. With good help after birth, you should be able to get your baby well latched to your breast.

Deeply buried nipples, on the other hand, are likely to need help during pregnancy to become more graspable. One method is to stretch the skin of the areola enough to enable the nipple to protrude. You can put your two forefingers on either side of your nipple at the base and gently push your fingers apart. Repeat this procedure all around your nipple, pulling any adhesions loose. You may have to do this several times every day to notice a difference.

If this technique is less effective than it needs to be to develop a nipple that will fit into a new baby's mouth, you might try wearing a breast shell inside a bra that is one size larger than what you would ordinarily wear. When this device is worn inside a bra, it puts gentle pressure on the areola, gradually stretching your nipple. Wear the shell for a few hours each day, progressively increasing the amount of time you wear it, if you can do this without discomfort. You should wash the breast shells daily if you use this technique.

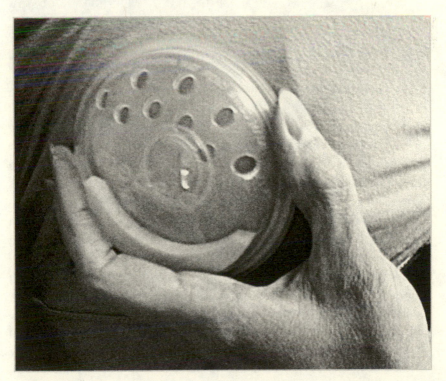

Breast shell

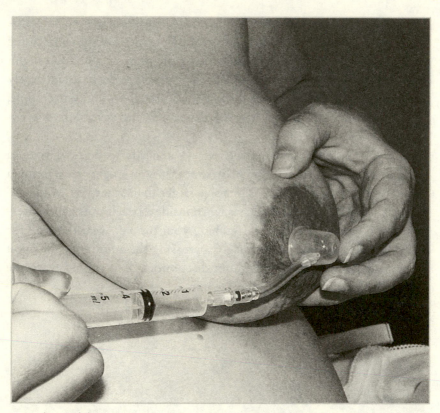

A chopped-down syringe can coax out an inverted nipple.

A third method involves using a disposable syringe (10 ml in size or—if your nipples are quite large—20 ml). Remove the piston from the syringe and cut off the nozzle with a sharp knife. Reinsert the piston in the cut end of the barrel. Put the smooth end of the syringe over your nipple and gently pull the piston for a few seconds to lengthen your nipple. Once you have loosened any adhesions, grasp your nipple between your thumb and forefinger and gently roll your nipple while stretching it outward to lengthen it.

You can also buy a device called the Evert-it nipple enhancer, which is available on the La Leche League website.

Before any implements such as those mentioned above were available, people used to "redesign" severely inverted nipples by using an empty tobacco pipe and a husband. I remember a nineteenth-century medical text that suggested if the husband couldn't or wouldn't help, "an intelligent serving maid" would suffice.

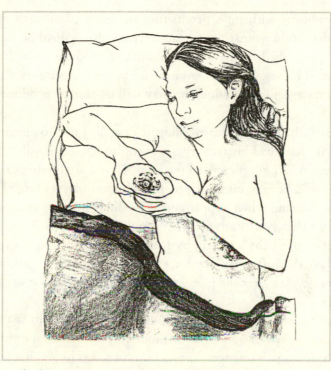

This breast squeeze can reduce swelling in pregnancy or engorgement while nursing.

Dealing with Discomfort from Swollen Breasts During Pregnancy

Some women with extremely large breasts experience so much breast swelling during pregnancy that they long for relief. In cases like this, it often helps to apply the kind of manual pressure illustrated in this drawing. This is best done when you are lying on your back.

Previous Breast Surgery

There is no way to be sure whether previous breast surgery will hinder your ability to produce milk or to allow it to flow from your breast. You will know only if you try. In general, minor surgeries such as a lump removal or a biopsy should not have a negative effect on lactation. Cosmetic surgeries, whether for breast reduction or augmentation, can cause problems with milk production or release, but such problems vary widely from woman to woman and may also depend on the type of surgery performed. Some women naturally produce enough milk to feed several babies. If such a woman has had breast surgery that interferes with her letdown reflex, she may still be able to produce enough milk to feed one baby.

Given the benefits of breastfeeding, it's usually good to plan to breastfeed if you have had breast surgery, even though it's possible that you may need to give supplemental feedings. If you are unable to produce enough milk, keep in mind that many babies value suckling enough to continue nursing when supplemental feedings become necessary. Do make sure that your midwife or physician is aware of your surgery, and check your baby's weight by four days after birth and every couple of days thereafter. By day six, your baby should be gaining about an ounce per day after the initial normal weight loss (no more than ten percent).

Breast-reduction surgery may involve the removal of breast tissue or liposuction—the removal of fat without surgical removal of breast tissue. If your surgery involved liposuction only, it is likely that your milk ducts and nerves were not cut, so your ability to produce and release milk should not be affected. Most kinds of breast-reduction surgeries, however, do involve cutting at least some of the milk ducts and nerves, producing a kind of damage that can interfere with the letdown reflex. Generally speaking, the more tissue that is removed, the greater the chance that supplemental feeding will be necessary. If you had reduction surgery and you still retain some feeling in your areola, there is a good chance that you can breastfeed exclusively. When there is no sensation left at all, your letdown reflex is less likely to function as it should, since this reflex depends upon the messages that travel from your nipple and areola to your brain to trigger milk production and release. Most of the sensation that is going to return following surgery will take place within two years. All this said, there have been some reported cases of women whose milk ducts healed and functioned fully after being cut during surgery. If you have had incisions around your areolae, I recommend that you rent an automatic electric breast pump and begin using it about three days after birth. Pump both breasts for four to five minutes after each feed to stimulate greater milk production.

It may take a week or two to build up a good supply, but the only way to find out if this will work for you is to try it.

I have worked both with women who could breastfeed exclusively following breast-reduction surgery and those who needed to supplement. One woman I know was able to nurse her first baby, because she had the extra time she needed in order to do it (her letdown reflex was damaged but not destroyed). When she gave birth to her second child less than eighteen months later, though, she was unable to spend as many hours nursing as the baby required, since doing so would have meant neglecting her older baby—who still needed some undivided attention. The mother would have preferred to breastfeed exclusively, but she ended up resorting to supplementary feedings for her younger baby.

For more advice on breastfeeding after breast-reduction surgery, I recommend Diana West's *Defining Your Own Success: Breastfeeding After Breast-Reduction Surgery*. Her website (www.bfar.org) is another good resource.

Breast-augmentation surgery involves the use of either silicone- or saline-filled implants. These may be inserted through an incision around the areola or an incision in the fold under the breast, near the armpits. Again, the extent of the damage is related to the location of the incisions. If the incisions were made around the areola, it is possible that milk ducts or nerves were damaged by the surgery. On the other hand, if your scars are in the folds under the breast or near the armpits, it is likely that your implants were inserted *behind* your milk ducts. If neither your ducts nor your nerves were cut, your ability to suckle your baby is likely to be unaffected. About half of women with this type of surgery are able to fully nurse their babies, according to one study.[1]

Augmentation surgery always causes scarring inside the breast, whichever way the surgery is done, and it can sometimes cause discomfort during nursing or put pressure on the milk-producing glands, reducing the milk supply. Another effect of the surgery is that your nipples may be more or less sensitive than normal.

Some mothers wonder if their milk might be contaminated by the presence of their silicone implants. In the 1990s, a small study of six breastfed babies claimed that these implants might cause problems with swallowing. The group that offered this hypothesis was heavily criticized, mainly for how its subjects were chosen.[2] Over the next few years, several larger studies with better methodology found no connection between the presence of silicone implants and esophageal disorders in breastfed babies.[3-5] Both the American Academy of Pediatrics' Committee on Drugs and La Leche League International recommend that mothers with implants should breastfeed their babies exclusively if possible.

What Do You Really Need to Buy?

Buying a Sling

There are a few things that you will need to buy if you are planning on exclusively breastfeeding your baby. One product that I would recommend is a good sling so you can tie your baby close to your body between feedings. Many first-time mothers are surprised by how much their newborns like to be held during the first month or two, even when their bellies are full. A sling will allow you to satisfy your baby's need to be close to you without taking away your mobility. Dads can use these slings too.

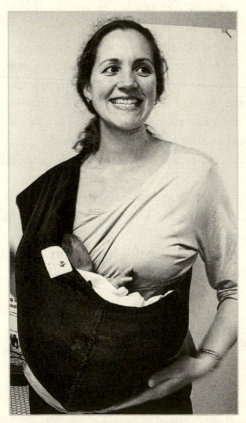
Wearing your baby in a sling frees your hands while calming your baby.

When you shop for a sling, keep in mind that you'll want one that can work as well for a newborn as it can for a two-year-old. I would recommend that you avoid the kind that has a covered metal frame; chances are high that your baby will find this as uncomfortable as you do. The soft cloth sling that cups your baby's body will allow the kind of contact between you and your baby that he craves, and it will also permit breastfeeding. Another advantage of this kind is its washability.

Buying a Nursing Bra

You will need to buy good nursing bras during your pregnancy. Buying the right bra for nursing can be a little tricky, since your breasts will go through more than one change in size after you give birth. For that reason, I recommend that you buy just one or two that aren't very expensive for early use until your breasts settle down to the size they will be for the next several months. Then you can buy about three of the style and size that works best for you. This size change may take a couple of weeks.

Choose one cup size larger than is comfortable during pregnancy and possibly one size larger than your usual number, especially if you're already using the loosest fastening. Take enough time in the fitting room to notice if you can uncover one breast without tightening the fabric on any part of your other breast, since such pressure could cause a blocked milk duct, which could lead to mastitis. You should not buy any bra that leaves marks on your shoulders or any other area, as a too-tight bra can also cause a blocked duct. For this same reason, you should avoid a bra with plastic-lined cups or underwires.

Look for a style that allows you to drop a flap at a time with one hand without having to look. All-cotton is the best choice for fabric, because most synthetic fabrics trap moisture next to your skin (your nipples should be dry between feedings). Adjustable, wide nonelastic straps are best. If your breasts are really heavy, you might like slightly padded straps as well.

If your breasts are small, you may not even need a bra for support. You might choose a simple stretch bra (not too tight), that can hold absorbent breast pads if you are prone to leaking. This kind of bra can be pulled up for nursing.

If you need to return to your outside job, you might find a hands-free bra to be useful. This kind of bra is worn only while pumping. It's a bustier that is worn over your regular nursing bra. If you plan to give birth at a hospital or birth center, be sure that in addition to a nursing bra(s) you buy a nightgown or pajama top that has an opening that will work for breastfeeding.

How Necessary Is a Breast Pump?

If you plan to be at home with your baby for the first year or so of life, you can most likely do without a breast pump—unless you are faced with circumstances that require you to travel without your baby. If you have an outside job that you'll be returning to after giving birth, see Chapter 8 for advice on buying breast pumps and for information on other preparations that can help you to continue breastfeeding once you return to your job.

Make Your Home Comfortable

While you are still pregnant, it's a good idea to create at least one good place in your home for nursing. You'll want a comfortable chair, a way to prop your feet up, a table within reach where you can put a large drink, a snack, a television remote, or a phone—whatever you might need while you are suckling your baby. Many women enjoy listening to audio books while they are nursing, so it might be a good idea to buy some or check some out from the library.

Lullabies

Learn some lullabies while you are pregnant, if you don't already have some favorites. You don't have to be a great singer to sing to your baby. Your baby won't know the difference and will appreciate whatever you do. The advantage of singing to your baby during pregnancy is that he will learn the songs while he's still in the womb and will respond to them well after birth. A great lullaby is a way of calming yourself and your baby at the same time, and a calm baby usually nurses the best.

A French friend taught me a captivating lullaby called "Bébé Lune," which she began singing to her son when he was a newborn. When he was nine, she would still sing it to him at bedtime, and he found it such a powerful sleep inducer that he would beg her not to sing it yet when he wanted to hear another story. Every great lullaby has a slow, calm rhythm.

Dietary Needs

Developing a good relationship with food is an important part of preparing for a healthy pregnancy and breastfeeding experience. Inadequate nutrition during pregnancy and the nursing period can result in your being unnecessarily fatigued and less resistant to illness. Remember that, in general, eating a well-balanced and varied diet of foods is better than relying on supplements to meet your nutritional needs and those of your growing baby. It's less expensive as well.

Your diet should include fresh vegetables and fruits, protein- and calcium-rich foods, and whole grains or cereals. Whole-grain crackers, nuts, cheese, yogurt, fresh fruits, sprouts, and raw vegetables are some of the nutritious foods that you might want on your list.

It's best to eat food and only food—that is, eat foods that are as close as possible to their natural state, and keep away as much as possible from highly processed products that contain chemical additives such as preservatives, artificial colorings, and artificial sweeteners. The same goes for what you drink. If you are addicted to sweet beverages, try cutting down or even swearing off them during pregnancy and breast-feeding, drinking more water and noncaffeinated teas instead. Sugar adds calories without nutrition, and chemical sweeteners come with unpleasant side effects such as dizziness, memory loss, and even weight gain. Have a sweet treat now and then (sugar or honey is preferable to artificial sweeteners), but remember that most of the calories you consume should directly benefit you and your baby.

It's good to know that grilling, steaming, boiling, roasting, and baking are ways to heat and cook foods without adding excess calories of fat. Fried foods, on the other hand, add many calories without providing added nutritional benefit.

Now let's examine the elements you will need most from your diet to ensure that you have a healthy pregnancy and are prepared for nursing.

Protein-rich foods include fish, poultry, eggs, meat, dairy products, legumes (dried beans of various types), tofu, and nuts. You need these to nourish not only your own body but your baby's as well, whether you are pregnant or nursing. High-protein foods tend to "stick to your ribs" longer than grains, fruits, or vegetables do. If you are concerned about gaining weight too fast (or not losing as quickly as you'd like while you nurse), continue to eat protein-rich foods, fruits, vegetables, and whole grains, and reduce the amount of sweet foods you eat. Remember that one of the symptoms of inadequate protein intake is a strong craving for sweets. If your budget is tight, take note that legumes and tofu cost less than meat and dairy products and are just as nourishing.

Vitamin- and mineral-rich foods include green vegetables such as green beans, Swiss chard, kale, spinach, bok choy, different kinds of lettuce, green peppers, and collards, and yellow vegetables such as sweet potatoes, yams, carrots, and red and yellow peppers. Sprouts are another excellent choice, and finely chopped cabbage or kale can be a tasty addition to a fresh salad. If you include a good variety of these foods in your daily diet, you should not need to add supplements.

You are an exception to this rule if you are a vegetarian who eats no eggs or dairy products. You *will* need to supplement vitamin B12, as a deficiency in this important vitamin can result in pernicious anemia, which can cause serious fatigue, miscarriage, and premature birth. The recommended amount is about three to four milligrams per day. Look for this supplement at a food store, or look for "nutritional yeast" (*Saccharomyces cerevisiae*, a food yeast grown in a molasses solution). Yellow or gold in color from its riboflavin content, it is easily digestible and tasty. Besides containing plenty of B12, it also contains all of the essential amino acids. It is not the same as brewer's yeast or torula yeast.

Calcium-rich foods include dairy products, dark-green leafy vegetables, whole grains, legumes, tofu, blackstrap molasses, carrot juice, oats, beets, nuts, and sesame seeds—all of which contain several other nutritionally important components as well. If you like fish, try eating mackerel, salmon, and sardines, all of which are good sources of calcium. Taking calcium supplements during pregnancy or while nursing will not affect calcium levels in your milk, so it is safe to stick to four servings of calcium-containing foods per day instead of taking supplements.[6–7] Contrary to popular belief, breastfeeding does not increase your risk of osteoporosis in later life. Although bone density decreases slightly during the nursing period, once you wean, your body returns to prepregnancy bone-density levels. The traditional diets of Japan and China, where women have the lowest rates of osteoporosis in the world, include lots of dark-green vegetables and almost no dairy products. All this said, some pregnant women do experience insomnia or leg cramps during the night, which indicates that they should increase their calcium intake, either by adding calcium-rich snacks or taking a calcium supplement. If you choose the latter, I recommend that you get a calcium lactate supplement, preferably one that is blended with magnesium at a 2:1 ratio (calcium to magnesium). Take it just before bedtime, as calcium is more readily absorbed while you sleep.

Iron-rich foods are good to eat while you are pregnant or nursing. Sources include dark molasses, egg yolk, whole grains, legumes, leafy vegetables, raisins, prunes, brewer's yeast, liver, and nuts. The normal increase in your blood volume during the second trimester of pregnancy may make your hemoglobin and hematocrit levels drop a bit. If your iron stores are low enough during pregnancy or after birth to make you feel fatigued and listless, six to eight alfalfa tablets per day can improve them quickly, and these tablets also seem to have a beneficial effect on milk production. If you do take an iron supplement, choose ferrous citrate or ferrous gluconate instead of ferrous sulfate, as these forms are more easily utilized and less likely to cause constipation or liver damage.

Iron is similar to calcium in that the iron levels in your milk are not affected by the amount of iron you consume in your diet or by supplementation. Full-term babies are born with ample iron stores, which normally last them well past the age of six months. At that time they are usually ready to eat some solid foods as they continue to nurse. Solid foods plus the iron in your milk can supply the dietary iron your baby needs from then on. A premature baby, on the other hand, may need iron supplementation before starting solid foods, since his iron stores will be lower at birth than those of a full-term baby.

Vitamin D is another important component of breast milk, entering your body through dietary sources and exposure to sunlight. Most babies who get only breast milk will not be at risk for developing rickets, a disease that can result from vitamin D deficiency, because the vitamin D in mother's milk plus the amount they themselves synthesize from sunlight exposure is sufficient to prevent it. It is possible, however, that dark-skinned women whose skin is seldom exposed to sunlight may have lower-than-desirable vitamin D levels when they begin their pregnancies. (The more pigmentation in skin, the more exposure to sunlight is necessary to get the same amount of vitamin D synthesis.) If you and your baby are dark-skinned and you are nursing exclusively, you should give him several minutes per day of exposure to sunlight on as much skin area as possible. If your own vitamin D intake is low and there is no way to make sure that your dark-skinned baby is regularly exposed to sunlight (maybe you avoid vitamin-D-supplemented dairy products and rarely get sunlight on your skin because of sunscreen or clothes that cover your skin), your pediatrician may recommend supplementation of 5 to 7.5 mcg of vitamin D per day for him. To combat your own low vitamin D levels, you may want to supplement with about 1,000 IU per day. However, it's not good to take too much vitamin D, as it can cause kidney stones.

Salt your food to taste, as salt is necessary for a normal pregnancy. If you like spicy flavors, there is no reason to avoid them during pregnancy or while nursing. The flavor of your milk will vary according to what you eat, but most babies tolerate these flavor changes without complaints. That said, there are babies who occasionally become cranky or show symptoms of temporary digestive upset when their mothers eat dairy products, citrus fruits and juice, cabbage, broccoli, cauliflower, garlic, onion, cinnamon, or chocolate. Signs that a baby isn't tolerating a food well include fussiness at the breast, redness around the anus, greenish poop, vomiting, and sudden refusal to nurse.

Dietary supplements, especially DHA supplements, are heavily marketed to breastfeeding mothers. Docosahexaenoic acid (DHA) is an omega-3 fatty acid found in breast milk and certain other natural sources such as cold water, oily fish, algae, pumpkin seeds, flax seeds, walnuts, soy beans, navy beans, and kidney beans. Although there is no definitive research pointing to a need for breastfeeding mothers to supplement with DHA to improve their milk, a common theme of the marketing campaigns has been that taking such supplements is a way of boosting babies' intelligence.

Caffeine deserves a special mention, since you are likely to receive so many mixed messages about it. Many babies can tolerate their mother's intake of a limited amount of caffeine without becoming irritable or cranky. Some babies, however, are more sensitive to their mother's caffeine consumption and exhibit colicky symptoms. If you suspect that there might be a connection between your caffeine intake and fussiness in your baby, limit or eliminate caffeine and see if he settles down over the next two days or so. Be aware that coffee, many iced and hot teas, colas, some soft drinks, and several over-the-counter pain-relief medications are all sources of caffeine (Excedrin, Midol, and Anacin are examples). If your caffeine intake is relatively high, an abrupt elimination of all caffeine is not a good idea, as your reward may be a withdrawal headache. Substitution of a decaffeinated drink (like decaf coffees and teas) may make it easier for you to limit caffeine in your diet.

Getting to a Healthy Pregnancy Weight

A normal weight gain during pregnancy ranges between 25 and 40 pounds (11 to 18 kg), depending upon your metabolism and activity level. Please don't be disappointed just after giving birth if you don't lose all your "baby weight" immediately. Almost no one does. The reason for this is that the weight of your baby, placenta, and amniotic fluid (the amount to be lost at birth) amounts to a little more than half of the normal pregnancy weight gain. More than forty percent of total weight gain is due to your increased blood supply, your heavier uterus and breasts, and some fat stores that will gradually melt off your thighs and hips as you nurse your newborn. This weight is best lost gradually over several weeks or even months after birth. It is never a good idea to go on a weight-loss diet while pregnant or nursing, as doing so can have negative effects on your health. Stay away from weight-loss drugs and "water" pills (also called diuretics), as these can be dangerous and even reduce your milk supply.

If you are not already in the habit of counting calories, it is not necessary to do so. A good general rule is to eat until your hunger is satisfied. Pregnant and nursing women often find that eating smaller, more-frequent meals works better for them than keeping to a three-meal-a-day plan. If you are accustomed to counting calories, the approximate number you'll need per day (while pregnant or lactating) is about 2,200. Don't eat less than 1,800 calories per day, especially if you are an active person.

3

How Birth Practices

Affect Breastfeeding

I hope the preceding chapters have laid to rest any lingering doubts you may have had about your body's innate ability to produce milk for your baby in the days following birth. Your body works as well as the bodies of your ancestors, almost none of whom had access to any sort of infant-feeding or birth technology. Even though your culture may make you feel uneasy about breastfeeding (depending upon where you live), you are still part of a species that has existed successfully on this planet for at least two thousand generations and has, for the most part, depended upon artificial feeding of its young for little more than half a century. There's another blessing—your baby's body has the same level of innate wisdom that yours does and is programmed with similarly awesome survival features.

At the same time, it's important to recognize that your ability to produce the appropriate hormones at the necessary times during and after birth to facilitate a great start in breastfeeding depends a good deal—

perhaps more than you might realize—upon the environment in which you give birth and the birth practices commonly used there. Wherever you choose to give birth, make sure that it is the type of environment that takes account of the needs of you and your baby just after birth, facilitates breastfeeding by giving you and your baby uninterrupted time to relate with each other (if all is well with you and your baby), and provides you with the kind of support that helps you solve any problems that you might meet as you and your baby begin this new phase of your life together.

Choosing where and how you will give birth is one of the most important preparations you can make for a good breastfeeding experience. I have been in hospitals in which the most commonly performed birth practices combined to almost rule out breastfeeding for most women, and I have been in others where nearly one hundred percent of the women who gave birth were breastfeeding their babies when they left the hospital. In this chapter, I'll present the best evidence I can to help you make educated decisions about birth choices that may affect your success in breastfeeding. These include the possibility of hiring a doula, the positions that you may assume in labor and birth, your ability to move around freely during labor, strategies for dealing with pain during labor, how much skin-to-skin contact you can have with your baby during the first half hour to hour following birth, and the amount of contact you have with your baby during a hospital stay.

I'll also discuss how common obstacles to breastfeeding—such as early separation from your baby, an epidural, a vacuum extraction, forceps delivery, or a cesarean—can be overcome. None of the above circumstances will make your breastfeeding experience any easier, but lots of women who have had these interventions are able to breastfeed. If you have had one or more birth interventions, though, you may have to be extra persistent to continue nursing and you may need the help of a dedicated lactation consultant—not just while you are at the hospital but sometimes even after you return home. Fortunately, most hospitals have lactation consultants available, and others specialize in the counseling that many women need during the first weeks of breastfeeding. If you do have trouble with nursing after birth interventions, you must not get too frustrated and discouraged—remember that you and your baby are genetically hardwired to make nursing work and that many mothers have overcome similar obstacles.

In my own first breastfeeding experience, my daughter was born by a mandatory forceps extraction shortly after I had been given a dose of Demerol (meperidine) followed by a caudal anesthesia, which temporarily paralyzed and numbed me from the waist down. I hadn't wanted either form of pain medication, so these interventions came as a rude shock to me. The caudal meant that I was warned not to lift my head even an inch for the next twelve to fourteen hours, lest I get a spinal headache that might stay with me for three months. Another nonnegotiable item was the chance to see my baby before she was twenty-four hours old. Despite these gross interventions (there was an episiotomy too), my daughter latched on to my breast as soon as I cuddled her close enough to make it possible. It was sheer good luck that she was brought to me at a time when she was wide awake and alert and not too full of infant formula to keep her from being interested in nursing. I had the additional good fortune to have a roommate who gave birth shortly before I did, and she was one of the mere twenty percent of women in the mid-1960s who decided to breastfeed. I just imitated her. I have no way of knowing whether I would have been successful without her good example.

Doulas Improve Birth Outcomes, Breastfeeding, and Mothering

Doulas are trained and experienced in giving continuous emotional and physical help throughout labor. In times past, it was common knowledge that it was easier for women to go through labor and give birth if they were provided with the continuous presence and kindly (nonmedical) advice of female friends or relatives. Nowadays, more and more women are turning to doulas for help during labor. Physicians, midwives, and nurses are hard-pressed to give this kind of attention, since they are typically required to look after several different women on any given day and cannot be continuously present in one woman's labor room. Evidence for the positive impact of the presence of a supportive relative, midwife, nurse, or doula at the side of a laboring woman is quite strong: Many studies have found that women with labor support had shorter labors and much less need for pain medication, intravenous oxytocin augmentation, forceps, vacuum extraction, and cesarean section than women who labored without this care.[1-3] Not surprisingly, the greater chance you have of a shorter, less exhausting, undisturbed labor and birth, the greater will be your ability to enjoy the important time after birth when nature intends that you bond with and begin to breast-feed your baby. On average, having a doula with you during labor halves the time of labor as well as the likelihood of having a cesarean.

If you think you can't afford to hire a doula, please talk to your physician or midwife about whether there is a volunteer doula service in your area. If there isn't, maybe one of your girlfriends or relatives would like the idea of being your companion during labor and birth. If she is sympathetic and does some reading about what a doula does, she may save you a lot of unnecessary stress during labor.[4] Whether she has breastfeeding expertise or not (it's a good idea to find out), her help during labor may prove invaluable.

Any midwife who has assisted out-of-hospital births over a period of years has encountered cases in which labor was hampered by the presence of too many well-meaning observers. This is most likely to occur during the opening phase of labor, which might be meaningfully described as the entry to a trance state. At this time, much depends upon the behavior of everyone present. Though no one who attends your birth will want to make your labor any harder, some family members may be compassionate enough to know how to make their presence helpful, and others may prove to be harmful distractions, slowing your labor unintentionally. Depending upon your comfort level, it may make you anxious to have even two or three companions during birth (for instance, if you grew up in a family in which the bathroom door was always locked and bodily functions were never discussed). In general, it's better not to allow people to be with you during labor and birth unless you are really certain that their presence is going to be valuable to you. A sensitive doula can be helpful in getting any well-meaning but inhibitory people out of your immediate presence during labor. This will probably be easier for her to do than for you or your partner, since she does not have a personal relationship with your guests. For example, if some of the people in the room where you'll be laboring are texting or watching television to pass the time, your doula may suggest that they do this in another room, since it is unlikely that their presence is helping you.

It's far better to have a doula than to write out a birth plan, because labor rarely proceeds according to anyone's plan.

Freedom to Choose Maternal Position
in Labor Helps Breastfeeding

If you have ever watched different kinds of mammals in labor, whether in real time or in a video or film, you probably noticed how much they move. Among land mammals, there is much swaying of the hips, shifting of weight from foot to foot, and other movement that may seem purposeless to the uninitiated. Marine mammals tend to be active in labor as well. I remember watching a video of a pregnant killer whale who swam in energetic spirals in the water, twisting and turning to help her baby find her way out. There are reasons for these movements—sometimes the baby is not in the best position to exit the womb and needs to shift in relation to its mother's body. For instance, if a mare's foal is malpositioned for birth (the foal's spine is near the mare's belly instead of near her spine), the mare will lie on the ground and throw her entire body back and forth to help her baby rotate to a more favorable position. The same thing can happen in humans. Midwives know that when a woman stays in the same posture throughout labor and her baby is poorly positioned, the baby is unlikely to spontaneously move into a better position for birth. On the other hand, if the woman moves from lying down on a bed to her hands and knees, changing positions frequently, she can sometimes help the baby roll a full 180 degrees. This might prevent an unnecessary C-section.

Many women don't realize this, but labor pain is accentuated by having enforced stationary positions throughout labor. According to Listening to Mothers II (a nationwide survey of 1,600 U.S. women, each of whom gave birth to a single child in 2005), two-thirds of U.S. women now get their main information about childbirth from television rather than from childbirth-education classes. This means that most of the births they have seen were to women on epidurals lying still during labor, waiting for it all to be over. Seeing this kind of birth over and over again causes a subconscious imprint on the mind, and many women develop enough fear of the pains of childbirth that they block the messages their bodies give them about other positions they might take in labor. Others may simply fear diverging from the norm.

A woman in the first stage of labor may find it beneficial to try several upright positions: standing, perhaps leaning on a counter or tray table; slow dancing with her partner; sitting while leaning forward or propped up with pillows; squatting; or sitting in a rocking chair. Sometimes one position suffices, but laboring women usually like to change from one position to another as labor progresses. One of the most effective labors I ever witnessed was that of a first-time mother giving birth to a very large baby. She moved through the first part of labor very efficiently by belly-dancing while putting as much of her weight as possible on a long staff she was holding to steady herself. She then pushed her baby out while leaning on the bed in a kneeling position.

A woman's position during labor and birth may affect her ability to breastfeed in a couple of ways. Dr. Roberto Caldeyro-Barcia, an Uruguayan obstetrician, was one of the first to scientifically investigate the effects of maternal position on labor. In 1979 he published a study now regarded as a classic, which demonstrated that mothers in a "vertical" position had thirty-six percent shorter opening stages of labor than "horizontal" women; the "vertical" women also reported less pain than the "horizontals." Walking helped labor progress as well, because it brought the pressure of the baby's head against the cervix, helping it to thin and open. And the "vertical" mothers' babies' heads were less apt to be extremely molded just after birth, indicating a somewhat smoother passage through the mother's birth canal. Equally important, the babies of women who gave birth in upright positions had less fetal distress at birth.[5] These factors all increase the chances that a woman will have a good early breastfeeding experience.

Dr. Caldeyro-Barcia's research also showed that requiring mothers to give birth lying flat on their backs, with their legs in stirrups, can compress the mothers' major blood vessels, preventing adequate oxygenated blood from flowing to their babies. Women who are mobile during labor are much less likely to face this problem.

The policy at some hospitals is that there should be electronic fetal monitoring throughout labor, which usually means laboring women are confined to bed. You should be aware, though, that good research shows that listening intermittently to the baby's heart rate with a handheld Doppler is an equally effective way to monitor the baby's condition. Many hospitals require a twenty-minute period of continuous monitoring, which, if favorable, can be followed by intermittent monitoring with the handheld device.

Eating and Drinking During Labor

The practice of prohibiting mothers from eating and drinking during labor began in the United States during the 1940s, when a considerable proportion of vaginal births happened with the mother under a general anesthesia. This type of anesthesia causes nausea, and the danger it introduced was of women vomiting while unconscious and then inhaling some of the contents of the stomach. This complication could potentially lead to a fatal form of pneumonia.

By the second half of the twentieth century, it had become rare for women to give birth under general anesthesia. The newer forms of anesthesia (epidural and spinal) no longer made women unconscious or nauseous. Given these new conditions, it would have made sense to relax the routine prohibition of eating and drinking during labor, which is, after all, very hard work for most women—work that requires that energy be replenished in some fashion when it lasts more than seven or eight hours. Though some women will indeed be able to give birth within that amount of time, many more will not—especially if they are restricted in their movements because of intravenous lines, electronic fetal-monitoring systems, and/or epidural anesthesia. My midwifery partners' and my experience with about 2,500 women over three and a half decades has shown us that many women can safely labor for twenty-four hours, or even more, as long as they are given some real sustenance if they desire it.

I recommend that you look for a maternity service that is flexible on the issue of eating and drinking during labor. If you can't find one, it's a good idea to eat a high-carbohydrate meal before leaving for the hospital. Conserving your energy is important, not just in terms of labor but also for breastfeeding. Eating and drinking as needed will help you be more alert for your first interaction with your baby.

The Effect of Pain Medication on Breastfeeding

If you are planning for your first baby and will be giving birth in a hospital, you may have already considered taking some form of pain-relieving medication during labor. Before you choose, it makes sense to consider the advantages and disadvantages of the medications you are likely to be offered if you are planning a vaginal birth. Knowing something about alternative methods of dealing with labor pain is also worth your consideration. There is no question that we all have to be grateful that we have medications to make procedures such as surgery painless. At the same time, the use of painkilling medications has always involved certain risks to mothers and babies that must be weighed for their use in labor, especially in the early part.

Epidural

The epidural is the best-known form of pain relief for labor in the United States. Even so, there can be some unwanted side effects associated with the epidural that may have some impact on getting a good start with breastfeeding.[6-8] Women who have epidurals must also be given intravenous fluids to counteract one of these side effects—drastically lowered maternal blood pressure, which, if left untreated, could cause a sudden drop in the baby's heart rate. The extra fluid from the IV may make your breasts more swollen than usual in the days following birth, which can make it difficult for your baby to latch on correctly.

Fever during labor is about five times more likely when an epidural is used than when the mother is unmedicated. The cause of this fever is not well understood, but it can mean a higher likelihood of your baby being stressed at birth, having poor muscle tone, needing resuscitation, and having seizures during the first few days, according to one large study.[9] Another drawback is that the epidural fever cannot be distinguished from a dangerous intrauterine infection unless the baby is evaluated. Such evaluation involves prolonged separation from the mother, possible admission to special care, painful tests, and usually antibiotic treatment until the test results are available. More than three times as many epidural babies were subjected to such evaluation as nonepidural babies, according to the above study. All of these interventions can interfere with the initiation of breastfeeding.

At the same time, a Toronto-based study published in 1999 found that in a hospital that strongly promotes breastfeeding, using epidurals for labor-pain relief does not interfere with breastfeeding success (the new mothers and babies were observed at six weeks following birth). An impressive seventy-two percent of the women who had epidurals were fully breastfeeding. However, thirty-six percent of the women in the study did have difficulty starting breastfeeding in the hospital because of sore nipples or difficulty latching.[10] It is highly probable that the results of this study may not be quite so easy to achieve outside of Toronto, which is home to one of the best breastfeeding clinic systems in the world, run under the guidance of Dr. Jack Newman, a well-known pediatrician-breastfeeding consultant and author. The good news that we can take from this report is that *with excellent breastfeeding support* over the first six weeks, a high proportion of women who have had epidurals can successfully breastfeed.

If you think there is a good chance that you might want an epidural, try to plan your care to take place in a hospital with nurses and lactation consultants who have a strong commitment to helping breastfeeding mothers get off to a good start.

Tranquilizers

Tranquilizers such as Valium, sedatives, and sleeping pills are all sometimes used to reduce anxiety and tension in laboring women, but they do cross the placenta and interfere with the baby's ability to breathe, to suckle, and to maintain a healthy muscle tension (tranquilized newborns tend to be limp). Such medications do not take away pain but rather increase pain tolerance. Nonetheless, they are still widely offered in U.S. hospitals.

Narcotics

Narcotics work on the central nervous system and would be effective at significantly reducing labor pain if they could be given in sufficient amounts. This is not possible, however, because doses high enough to lower labor pain are not considered safe for mother and baby. Demerol (meperidine) is still used as an analgesic in some U.S. maternity wards. A relatively small dose, given intravenously or by injection, can cause sleepiness, and it often causes nausea, vomiting, and a drop in blood pressure. Once administered, it crosses the placenta and reaches the baby in only two minutes. Don't expect a significant drop in pain.

Some studies have shown that babies exposed to Demerol and other narcotics have long-lasting effects when it comes to nursing.[11-12] Even if your baby is awake and appears to be alert, she may still have problems breastfeeding. A Swedish study of women given Demerol in labor found that twenty minutes after birth, more than half of the babies in the study were still too sedated to suckle at all. Eighteen percent had a disorganized suck. The authors found that the half-life of Demerol in a newborn ranges from thirteen to twenty-three hours.[13]

Stadol (generic name: butorphanol) and Nubain (nalbuphine) are other narcotics that are often used for labor analgesia. One study found that babies medicated with these narcotics were forty-four hours slower to establish breastfeeding than those who had no narcotics.[14]

Learn About Techniques for Reducing Pain

Before we leave the subject of labor pain, let's look at some of the often-overlooked nonmedical remedies that have proven effective for many women. As I've discussed, unrestricted movement during labor is a key way to decrease pain naturally. If you experience a lot of back pain, you may also try getting on your hands and knees. Another option is hydrotherapy, in the form of a shower or a warm, deep bath (if this is offered by the hospital you plan to use). Lots of women who get into water in early labor don't want to get out, because they find it so relaxing.

A physical-therapy birth ball is an excellent and inexpensive labor aid. You can use it to support your weight while kneeling, sitting, or standing during labor. Many mothers also find this ball useful after birth, as it provides you a great way to sit and hold your fussy baby while gently bouncing. The 65-cm-size ball is the one that is most widely used by women of average height. Choose a size larger or smaller, according to your own needs.

The detail of a famous sculpture by Bernini, "The Ecstasy of St. Teresa," shows the facial expression that I often see in the later stages of labor. Mind you, St. Teresa was not depicted giving birth; in fact, she was being visited by an angel, whose spiritual presence was so powerful that it put her into an ecstatic state. It's a good one to meditate on while you are still pregnant, as it's one of the expressions I most like to see on a woman in labor: The open jaw indicates surrender to the natural forces of labor. This goes with an optimal mix of birth hormones, which is the best preparation for an optimal mix of lactation hormones.

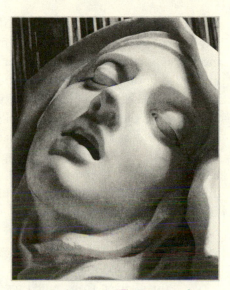

Detail of Bernini's "The Ecstasy of St. Teresa"

As part of your preparation for labor, I would recommend that you view the film *Orgasmic Birth,* as it offers you a chance to watch several women having unmedicated, ecstatic births.

The Sensitive Period Just After Birth

Farmers and those who raise animals have always known that there is a sensitive period just after birth. I first became aware of this concept at the age of nine, during the summer I spent at my aunt's farm. Besides raising milk cows and many other animals, my aunt Myra raised dogs, and at this particular time she had a bulldog with high needs. The bulldog gave birth to a litter of twelve pups in Aunt Myra's kitchen. I had never seen such young puppies before and immediately reached out to pick up one of the squirming litter. "Don't touch that pup!" shouted my usually soft-spoken aunt. I quickly withdrew my hand, stung by her strong reprimand. Aunt Myra then quietly explained that if I had contaminated the puppy with my smell, the mother might reject the puppy or even her whole litter. That incident made a deep impression on me; it provided my first understanding that maternal behavior, which I'd assumed was automatic in animals, could so easily be disrupted by well-meaning but ignorant human interference.

Michel Odent has pointed out that scientific research in the area of imprinting and attachment behavior began in the 1930s with Konrad

Lorenz's legendary experiment with ducks. Lorenz reported that one day he had placed himself between newly hatched ducklings and their mother and then imitated the mother's quacking sounds. The ducklings imprinted upon him and attached to him for the rest of their lives, following him as he walked around the garden.

Studies of the sensitive period in mammals have looked at various species, including rats, sheep, and goats. General findings have been that later separation of mother and young could be tolerated—that is, long-lasting bonds had been formed—as long as the separation did not occur during the sensitive period just after birth. However, in sheep, if the separation occurred just after birth and extended for four hours or so, half of the ewes simply wouldn't take care of their babies when they were reunited. In another study, when ewes were given epidurals in labor, they refused to take care of their lambs at all.

We humans seem to be much more adaptable than other mammals are when it comes to forming bonds with our newborn babies, even if we haven't had uninterrupted, skin-to-skin contact during the first hour following birth. All the same, many studies have made it clear how important this period can be to mothers who want to breastfeed their babies.

Delayed Cutting of the Umbilical Cord

You may be surprised to know how much the timing of umbilical-cord clamping can affect your breastfeeding experience. Despite the lack of any solid evidence that haste to cut the cord benefits baby or mother, immediate clamping of the umbilical cord is standard procedure in most U.S. hospitals, as if more placental blood would be detrimental to the newborn baby. This practice is probably a habit formed during a time when most babies were born to women under general anesthesia; many of these babies required immediate resuscitation, so their cords were clamped right away. Within the midwifery model of care, on the other hand, the tendency is to delay clamping and cutting the umbilical cord. The assumption is that a newborn will benefit from receiving the additional volume of blood that will be squeezed into her body in the first few minutes of life—as much as thirty percent of her total blood volume.

Certainly, nature has provided various designs among different species of mammals regarding when and how the placenta ceases to be a part of the fetus's or newborn's life-support system. Elephants and several other species of mammals, for example, have an umbilical cord that isn't long enough to enable the infant to be delivered until the cord breaks. There is usually a weak place in the cord, which snaps during the birth process, unless the placenta releases at the same time the infant is expelled. We can guess from this biological design that elephant calves probably don't need any more blood than the placenta transfers to them before the infant begins to move down the birth canal. But can we make the same assumption when it comes to human infants?

Judy Mercer, a U.S. nurse-midwife and professor of nursing, has been researching this subject for more than three decades. In 2006, her landmark study of early vs. late cord-clamping gained international attention by showing that a brief delay in clamping the cords of babies born before thirty-two weeks prevents—to a significant degree—bleeding in the brain and infections.[15] The National Institutes of Health found her data so promising that she was recently awarded $2 million to carry out a larger study that will look at the results of delayed clamping for full-term babies as well as after cesareans.

It is really odd that midwives and nurses who favor delayed clamping are in the position of having to prove that a few seconds' or minutes' delay has advantages to the baby. Midwives in out-of-hospital birth settings almost unanimously favor delayed cord-clamping—that is, waiting to clamp at least until pulsation of the cord has stopped. We usually keep the baby on approximately the same level as the mother, since we place her directly on her mother's abdomen just after birth as we wait for the placenta to be delivered.

One more important reason to negotiate with your physician or midwife for delayed cord-cutting is that, if your baby is still attached to your body in this way, any separation of the two of you will also be delayed. Your baby will have a much easier time adjusting to breathing and will be less likely to suffer from anemia if her cord is allowed to pulsate for several minutes after birth. (A vaginally born first twin may sometimes be an exception.)

A new trend called "cord blood banking" has been heavily marketed recently. What you may not realize is that such cord blood extraction requires immediate clamping of the cord and a rigorous process that can prove disruptive during the magical time just following birth.

Your Baby's Initial Evaluation

Step one for getting the best possible start at breastfeeding is for you and your baby to be as close together as possible just after birth. Skin-to-skin contact is especially important during the first hour, because of the hormonal changes taking place in you and your baby. These are magic moments for both of you. Biologically speaking, you two are still a unit and should be treated as such. Your baby's touch, movements, and "begging" sounds cause you to release the hormones that protect you against excessive blood loss, and your body's warmth protects your baby from loss of body heat. This is also a time for you to begin to learn your baby's cues—what her various sounds and movements mean.

Swedish researchers studied the benefits of skin-to-skin contact in the first hours after normal birth. They hypothesized that babies would cry less in their first hours of life if they had skin-to-skin contact with their mothers. The babies who were randomized to the skin-to-skin-contact group were compared with a group of babies who were similar in every other way except for being swaddled in double blankets and placed in a bed next to the mother. Not only did the skin-to-skin group cry less, they also had higher body temperatures and were less apt to experience low blood-sugar levels ninety minutes after birth than the swaddled group.[16] (A baby with a higher temperature is more likely to have the energy to latch on to the breast than one whose temperature is lower.) Nature didn't intend for mothers and their babies to be separated from each other after birth. In fact, immediate separation between mother and baby is one of the most efficient ways to make the initiation of breastfeeding *more* difficult.

Once your baby is born, your birth attendant will want to observe her condition. The initial evaluation can easily be done with her face-down on your abdomen or chest, since all that is necessary is the observation of her breathing, heart rate, muscle tone, reflex irritability, and skin color. The score given from this observation is called an Apgar score, named after Dr. Virginia Apgar, who invented the system several decades ago (as a way to assess babies exposed to medications).

Usually, within the first hour, your baby will be given a more thorough examination that checks for heart and lung function and looks for any problems that she might have, whether internal or external. It has long been the habit of most U.S. hospitals to do both this examination and the Apgar scoring on a special infant examination table under an infant warmer. However, both can be done just as well on your chest, and without immediate cutting of the umbilical cord. If done this way, the examination needn't upset your baby, and it will also give you a chance to talk with the examiner about what she is doing.

One of the most important recent studies on skin-to-skin contact, which, like the study mentioned on the previous page, was carried out in Sweden, describes the inborn behaviors that take place when mothers and newborns have uninterrupted contact. The researchers found that even painless procedures such as weighing, measuring, and bathing the newborn interfere with inborn feeding behavior.[17] Your baby's weight and height will not change during the first hours of life, so there should be no harm in delaying these procedures.

As for bathing (usually a routine hospital procedure just after birth), babies aren't born filthy. Blood, if present, may be gently wiped away, but the rest of what's on the baby's skin is conducive to the early initiation of breastfeeding, because the smell of amniotic fluid is an important stimulant to the nervous systems of both mother and newborn. The same principle should be applied to any attempt on the part of the nursing staff to wash your breasts. Two studies, prompted by scientists' awareness of the tendency for newborn mammals to find the smell of amniotic fluid attractive, considered the issue of smell in human infants. In one study, the mothers and babies were kept together, and the mothers washed one of their breasts. More than seventy percent of the babies moved toward the unwashed breast.[18] Another study separated babies from their mothers and placed them in a cot with a breast pad carrying their mothers' odor a few inches from their nose. The same babies were also given a clean breast pad. Not surprisingly, most of the babies moved toward the pad that smelled like their mother.[19]

Of course, circumstances sometimes require separation, as when a baby needs to be transferred to intensive care or a mother has more than normal blood loss. The point is that the mother and baby's need for each other should be recognized and fulfilled as much as possible throughout the hospital stay. Even if your baby has difficulties after birth and needs intensive care, it is usually possible for you to have a few minutes with her before she is transferred. If your baby is placed in intensive care in the hospital where you gave birth, you and other family members will be able to visit her there. Most intensive-care units have staff members whose job is to keep you informed about how your baby is doing and to reunite you with each other at the earliest opportunity.

If your baby is born prematurely or small for gestational age, you should know about the benefits of what is called the kangaroo-mother care model. First developed and described in Bogotá, Colombia, this low-tech method of care stabilizes premature babies through early and prolonged skin-to-skin contact in a kangaroo position between the mother's breasts. The method was initially promoted because of its cost-effectiveness, but subsequent research has shown that it is equally effective in countries with plenty of resources.[20] Besides all of the benefits that I have already discussed regarding early skin-to-skin contact, kangaroo-care premature babies are twice as likely to breastfeed, compared with incubator babies (eighty-two percent versus forty-five percent in one study). Mothers of kangaroo-care babies produced more milk, and their babies cried less and maintained their body temperatures better.

A California nurse, Carol Melcher, developed an ingenious "intervention" in the care of newborns that has significantly improved the initiation of breastfeeding in those hospitals that adopt it. Her method calls for new mothers to be encouraged to hold their newborns skin-to-skin during the first two hours following birth and as much as possible thereafter, unless there are specific medical problems with either that would rule this out. Nurses in hospitals that adopt her method postpone such interventions as the newborn bath, glucose sticks, footprinting, and eye treatments until after the first two hours, thus taking advantage of the strong suck reflex that a baby ordinarily has during the first hour or so following birth. If you plan to give birth in a hospital, you may want to find out if the nursing staff there is familiar with Melcher's "Breastfeeding Hospital Policy Recommendation #5." See Resources for information on how to access this policy recommendation. It is based upon very solid evidence.

Circumcision

Circumcision of newborn boys is a widespread practice in the United States that is usually performed before hospital discharge. With early discharge having become the norm, many babies are circumcised just a few hours after birth. Circumcision's impact on breastfeeding stems chiefly from its effect on the baby—though a local anesthetic may be used to partly numb the pain, this procedure can be both painful and extremely frightening for your baby. Newborns who undergo painful surgical procedures have high levels of stress hormones, which speed up their heart rates and suppress the high oxytocin levels that normally trigger their innate impulses to seek the breast.

There are no medical reasons compelling routine circumcision. The American Academy of Pediatrics recognized this in its 1999 statement: "Existing scientific evidence demonstrates potential medical benefits of newborn male circumcision; however, these data are not sufficient to recommend routine neonatal circumcision." The Canadian Paediatric Society made a similar statement in 2002, without adding the phrase about potential medical benefits, while the British Medical Association's 2003 statement was the most strongly worded of all: "The BMA does not believe that parental preference alone constitutes sufficient grounds for performing a surgical procedure on a child unable to express his own view. . . . Parental preference must be weighed in terms of the child's interests. . . . The BMA considers that the evidence concerning health benefit from non-therapeutic circumcision is insufficient for this alone to be a justification for doing it."

Because newborn circumcision was routine for so many decades in the United States, many parents-to-be lack information about what happens if there is no circumcision. Almost all newborn boys have tight foreskins during their first year of life. By the age of two, about half of boys' foreskins will have loosened from the head of the penis so that the foreskin can be retracted completely. (It's important that the foreskin not be forcibly retracted.) Once this is possible, it's an important part of hygiene that the foreskin be pulled back during a bath so that the accumulation of smegma can be removed. Only rarely does a circumcision become necessary because a foreskin cannot be retracted later in childhood or adulthood.

If you intend to breastfeed and you decide to go ahead with circumcision of your newborn boy, I recommend that you schedule it after your baby has experienced pleasure at your breast. Every lactation consultant I know has learned from experience that babies who undergo circumcision before they get a chance to suckle have more trouble taking the breast than those who are not frightened or subjected to a painful treatment during the first hours of life.

Immunizations

The same goes for immunizations. In some hospitals, it is routine to give all newborns immunizations very soon after birth, regardless of whether the babies have yet had a chance to nurse. Injections almost always hurt, and the experience of getting one soon after birth can cause a sensitive baby to become too tense and distrustful to feed at the breast for a while. When a twenty-four- or forty-eight-hour hospital stay is the norm, many babies have so many painful procedures within the first day of life that a chance at the breast is made unnecessarily difficult. The question then becomes: What justification is there for giving a newborn an immunization during the first day of life?

I can see only one situation when it would make sense to have an immunization on the first day of life: When a mother tests positive for hepatitis B, the vaccine should be given to the baby within twelve hours of birth. If possible, then, delay the shot until the half-day mark. The next immunizations can wait until your baby is two months old, so why not wait? These include the oral polio vaccine; the diphtheria, pertussis, and tetanus vaccine; and the hemophilus influenza B vaccine.

Rooming-In

Rooming-in means that you and your baby share the same room during your hospital stay instead of her being brought to you only at scheduled times. About sixty years ago, it became routine in U.S. hospitals for newborn babies to be taken away from their mothers and kept in a central nursery, where doctors and nurses could look after them. Dr. Marsden Wagner has called this practice the "biggest pediatric mistake of the last 100 years," referring to the frequent infectious epidemics in central nurseries, which caused significant loss of newborn lives.[21] Other problems with this setup are that it interferes with successful breastfeeding, deprives mothers of the chance to bond with their babies, creates multiple chances for mix-up of babies, and interferes with the development of mothers' self-confidence in caring for their newborns. It has to be said that these nurseries also led to a remarkable degree of ignorance about breastfeeding and its value for mothers and babies alike.

Starting life in a central nursery means little or no skin-to-skin contact between mother and baby, which results in less prolactin and therefore less milk than nature intended. It also creates opportunities, as well as temptations, for nurses to give your baby a pacifier or a feeding of infant formula, if they don't happen to be strong advocates for breastfeeding. Rooming-in, on the other hand, allows you to have as much skin-to-skin contact as possible with your baby. It means that you can breastfeed your baby as often as she would like—the way nature intended. Women in hunter–gatherer societies carry their babies next to their bodies and feed them many times a day once their milk supply is established.

The hospital practice of separating mothers and babies was not created to stop breastfeeding and bonding. That often may have been the result, but the practice began for other reasons. During the 1950s and 1960s, there were few medical studies that could be cited as evidence for keeping women and babies together, which made it difficult for anyone to argue in favor of it. At the same time, doctors and nurses received little or no education about the value of breastfeeding, and no one discussed the development of mothers' feelings for their babies and how this might be affected by hospital practices. This was also the era of general anesthesia and scopolamine, when a large proportion of U.S. women were so medicated in labor that they woke up unaware that their babies had been born. Many others—like me, for my first birth—were given a form of spinal anesthesia that made it necessary to avoid lifting their heads for half a day after giving birth if they didn't want to suffer a prolonged and severe spinal headache. Under these conditions, the central nursery became a necessity, because so many new mothers were unable to care for their babies during the first hours following birth. In many hospitals, a mother might see her baby only once during the first twenty-four hours and twice during the second day. No wonder so many people in this country began to think that breastfeeding didn't work!

During those decades, most North American women accepted the routine separation from their babies as medically necessary. I certainly did. No one suggested that I might want more access to my baby than the hospital was prepared to offer, and I never thought to ask what the rules about this were. I later found out that some nurseries three to four decades ago were so controlling that they forbade new mothers from unwrapping the blankets to have a closer look at their babies. Is it hard for you to believe that new mothers could be so easily intimidated as to obey such a crazy rule? Literally millions of women did, myself included.

I still remember how unprepared I felt when it was time to be discharged from the hospital, when my baby was five days old. During those few days, I had never once been trusted to change her diaper, dress her, or walk with her in my arms. The hospital policy of separation managed to convince me that the "experts" were better at caring for my daughter than I could ever be. That's a far cry from the kind of self-confidence I like to see in the new mothers in my care.

All this began to change during the 1960s and 1970s, when there was a resurgence of interest among women in being awake and aware during birth and in breastfeeding. At the same time, researchers in different parts of the world who were skeptical about the wisdom of routinely separating mothers and babies after birth began to carry out studies that looked at the unanticipated effects of early separation. One of the most intriguing of these early studies compared a test group of babies who were allowed skin-to-skin contact just after birth to a group of babies who didn't have such contact. The researchers noticed that in the skin-to-skin group, if the newborn babies were given enough uninterrupted time with their mothers and were left quietly on the mother's abdomen, gradually they crawled up to the mother's breast, found the nipple, and began to suckle. Fifteen out of sixteen babies were able to attach themselves in this way without any help—provided that the mother's labor was unmedicated and the babies had not been immediately taken away from their mothers for baths, vitamin K, weighing, or eye ointment. This was a revolutionary finding for wealthy countries, where it had become an article of faith among the medical profession that newborn humans did not have the skills exhibited by every other type of new-born mammal on the planet. A teaching video was later produced where these babies demonstrated to the world that they came out of the womb as well prepared as a puppy, a baby mouse, or a piglet (you can insert the name of any other mammal) to find the all-important nipple and to get down to the business of bringing in the milk supply that would sustain them during infancy.[22]

To summarize, here is a list of the tangible benefits of rooming-in that have been documented in scientific literature:

- Your milk production is likely to begin earlier.

- Your breasts are less likely to become engorged.

- Your baby is likely to have a faster weight gain.

- Your baby will be less likely to get jaundiced, because of quicker availability of your colostrum and milk. Practically speaking, this means less likelihood of your baby being separated from you for treatment of jaundice under bilirubin lights.

- Your baby is less likely to get an infection.

- Your baby will be more content and will cry less. Remember, she actually knows the difference between you and the nurses and prefers being held by you.

- You'll learn your baby's facial expressions and signals earlier.

- Your self-confidence as a mother will be enhanced.

- Caring for your baby from the very beginning will help you develop a stronger attachment to her. (Not everyone feels this strong bond right away, but solid evidence shows that close early contact helps it to develop.)

- You'll get more and better rest with rooming-in, because skin-to-skin contact with your baby will stimulate higher levels of the stress-reducing hormones oxytocin and prolactin in your system, and these hormones help you sleep better.

- You are less likely to experience postpartum depression.

Some hospitals offer so-called "modified rooming-in." This means that your baby spends most of the day with you in your room but is taken to the nursery each night. While modified rooming-in may sound good, and it is certainly preferable to a complete separation from your baby, it can present problems in getting started with breastfeeding. Babies tend to sleep a lot during the first two days of life, and some do not develop the kind of strong cry that might prompt the night nurses to bring her to you for a feeding. Some nurses might even consider it a kindness to you to give her a bottle during the night, letting you sleep. However well intentioned, this practice can delay your milk from coming in and work against a smooth start to breastfeeding. Additionally, the milk you give after midnight has a higher fat content, which your baby will miss out on if you are not able to give her a nighttime feeding. In view of this, I recommend that you take a tour of the hospital where you plan to give birth, to get a look at the facilities and see for yourself how that hospital defines rooming-in and how well this option is promoted. A relatively empty central nursery is a good sign that the staff regards rooming-in as the norm rather than an eccentric choice. A completely empty one is even better.

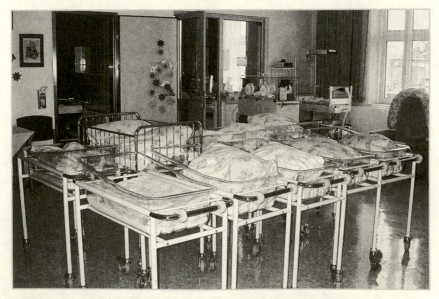

An empty central nursery in an Austrian hospital

Remember that it's important to know how full the nursery is during the night as well as during the day. Also, take note of the attitude of the person giving you the tour. Is the staff member enthusiastic about twenty-four-hour rooming-in? If modified rooming-in seems as far as the hospital is willing to go to accommodate breastfeeding, you may want to explore other options to see if you can find a more breastfeeding-friendly environment.

Despite the recommendations of the American Academy of Pediatrics, the choice of rooming-in is not available at all U.S. hospitals. The Listening to Mothers II survey (conducted by the Maternity Center Association) of 1,600 U.S. women who had given birth within the last two years found that only about sixty percent of the mothers interviewed had rooming-in.

Here are some questions that you can ask of your hospital to find out how much support the maternity care staff will give you and whether there will be any resistance to you having uninterrupted skin-to-skin contact with your baby during the first two hours and rooming-in for the rest of your hospital stay.

- Can you do the initial examination of my baby with her beside me?
- Can my baby be in the same room with me throughout my hospital stay?
- Is there any medical reason why my baby can't be with me?
- If there is any reason why my baby has to be taken from me, what care will be given to her?
- Who will be giving that care?
- When will my baby be brought back to me?
- Are you aware that I intend to breastfeed?
- Can my baby be given my breast milk during any separation from me?
- What kind of help will be available for me in learning how to breastfeed?
- Is kangaroo care possible if my baby is born prematurely?

Hospitals vary a lot as to whether rooming-in is a possibility for women whose babies are born prematurely.

In hospital units that strongly promote breastfeeding, premature babies are given skin-to-skin contact with their mothers as soon as they are able to breathe without a ventilator. I visited a neonatal unit in Prague, Czech Republic, in which rooming-in was the norm for premature babies as soon as they were breathing on their own. Their mothers were invited to begin to care for them as soon as they were off the ventilator. The pediatricians at this hospital were so convinced of the value of mother's milk for these tiny infants that they created a living unit large enough for about eight mothers. Each woman had a private sleeping space near a common kitchen and dining room. This arrangement, plus a generous paid maternity leave, allowed these babies to gain weight and strength at an optimal rate.

A neonatal unit in a children's hospital in northern Estonia was established in the late 1970s to provide medical and nursing care to newborn and premature babies and their mothers. The principles at this unit were twenty-four-hour care by the mother, minimal use of technology, and little contact between the baby and the medical and nursing staff. Each mother was given support by a team of doctors, nurses, psychologists, and massage therapists. She was taught to massage her baby every day and to keep notes on the baby's state of health. Every room was shared by two mothers, and there was a shared lounge area. The mothers were served meals in their rooms, so that they didn't have to leave their babies in order to eat. Fathers and other family members were encouraged to visit throughout the week. The medical director of the unit credited this approach with "considerable decreases in the number of infectious diseases," which meant less need for intravenous antibiotic therapy for the babies.[23]

The unit was able to compare the weight gain of babies who were cared for by their mothers with that of babies who were cared for by nurses (because these babies' mothers had decided to leave the job to them). The premature babies in the mother-care group showed significantly higher weight gains than the premature babies in the nurse-care group.

There is a trend toward twenty-four-hour rooming-in in most of Europe. I have been in several European hospitals in which the newborn nurseries were entirely empty at the time of my visit. By 2005, hospitals all across Sweden had phased out central nurseries by converting them into sitting rooms, dining rooms, or combination sitting–dining rooms for parents. Sweden has decided that the hospital has an important part to play in encouraging close relationships between parents and babies, as well as breastfeeding. They have dealt proactively with the possibility that misplaced sensitivity to negative staff attitudes rather than concern for their babies' needs might prevent some new mothers from rooming-in. Staff retraining did much to remove obstacles in the way of twenty-four-hour rooming-in.[24] One study provided what maternity policy-makers considered solid evidence that many new mothers will refrain from choosing rooming-in if they believe that the staff would prefer them to choose nursery care.

Here in the United States, there are varying attitudes about rooming-in among hospital staff members, probably because most hospital staffs have not been properly educated about how this arrangement can benefit both mother and baby. Some nurses who are unfamiliar with rooming-in may even leave obstetrics if rooming-in is phased in at their hospital. On a recent nursing forum on the Internet, one nurse said she was quitting because she couldn't believe the evidence of the value of rooming-in. She described it as "unsafe policies that put babies in danger." Another added, "...no dead babies yet. I can see so many things going wrong...aspiration, abducted babies, etc."[25] On the other side, there were some who saw for themselves how beneficial rooming-in can be: "We were very surprised to see that most [mothers] did not protest the change, as it gives them more time to learn how to care for their babies and ask questions while the baby is right there," said one nurse. Another, who did home follow-up care, said, "I think it is good to remember why keeping mothers and babies together is so important. I would see parents who hardly knew anything about their baby, and mothers with almost no milk production at post-delivery day four or five. I could tell who had spent a lot of time with their baby and who had not...."

Baby-Friendly Hospitals and the Ten Steps to Successful Breastfeeding

In 1991 the United Nations Children's Fund (UNICEF) and the World Health Organization (WHO) launched an international effort by developing a set of protocols for hospitals called the Ten Steps to Successful Breastfeeding.

The initiative was meant to begin a global effort to improve the effect of hospital maternity services on mothers' ability to initiate breastfeeding for their babies' best start in life. The ten steps are applicable to any birth setting, but they were formulated because of the strong evidence that many technology-driven hospital routines and procedures are a large factor in low rates of breastfeeding when mothers and babies are discharged from the hospital.

Step 1. Have a written breastfeeding policy that is routinely communicated to all health-care staff.

Step 2. Train all health-care staff in skills necessary to implement this policy.

Step 3. Inform all pregnant women about the benefits and management of breastfeeding.

Step 4. Help mothers initiate breastfeeding within half an hour of birth.

Step 5. Show mothers how to breastfeed, and how to maintain lactation even if they should be separated from their infants.

Step 6. Give newborn infants no food or drink other than breast milk, unless medically indicated. [Giving supplemental feedings in the first few days after birth is associated with an almost fourfold increase in the risk of being weaned by three months postpartum.]

Step 7. Practice rooming-in—that is, allow mothers and infants to remain together—twenty-four hours a day.*

Step 8. Encourage breastfeeding on demand.

Step 9. Give no artificial teats or pacifiers to breastfeeding infants.

Step 10. Foster the establishment of breastfeeding support groups and refer mothers to them on discharge from the hospital or clinic.

*Step 7 calls for twenty-four-hour rooming-in for all mothers, but in the U.S. this is interpreted as meaning all those who desire it—quite a step back from the usual definition of "all mothers."

Since 1991, the two organizations have promoted these steps around the world by designating hospitals that fulfill the ten steps as "Baby-Friendly."[26] Hospitals and birth centers that apply for Baby-Friendly recognition are evaluated according to their implementation of the Ten Steps to Successful Breastfeeding and their adherence to the WHO code.

To date, UNICEF has awarded this designation to about 20,000 hospitals in more than 150 countries. In many countries, mother's milk is considered such a vital national resource that the government requires every hospital to follow the ten steps.

Norway, for instance, had rates of breastfeeding initiation as low as those in the United States in the early 1970s, when only about a fifth of new mothers were breastfeeding their babies when they left the hospital. That country has completely changed its national policies by making sure that every Norwegian hospital in which babies are born is Baby-Friendly. At present, Norway leads the world in breastfeeding, with ninety-nine percent of Norwegian women breastfeeding at hospital discharge and more than eighty percent still breastfeeding when their babies are six months old.[27] In the United States in 2006, just seventy-seven percent of mothers were willing to try breastfeeding (but not exclusively) at discharge and only thirty-two percent were still nursing at six months.[28] According to a prominent Norwegian obstetrician–gynecologist and breastfeeding advocate, Dr. Gro Nylander, "At present it is more or less accepted in my country that it should be as unusual to feed animal milk to a newborn baby as it is to give human milk to newborn animals. . . ." And yet by far most Norwegian babies are born in hospitals. Clearly it is possible to design hospitals that combine the best of technology with enough restraint in its use to permit nearly every woman who wants to breastfeed to do so.

Baby-Friendly hospitals are not as easy to find in the United States as they should be. As of April 2009, only sixty-three U.S. hospitals in twenty-three states have been awarded Baby-Friendly status.[29] California, with eighteen such hospitals, has the greatest number, but most states don't have even one Baby-Friendly hospital.

So far, the lesson has been that Baby-Friendly status happens most often in countries in which the government provides effective direction, information, and resources to expedite the transition from hospital practices that are likely to interfere with the initiation and maintenance of breastfeeding to Baby-Friendly status as the norm. In these countries, breastfeeding rates rise significantly almost immediately.

Obstacles to the Baby-Friendly Hospital Initiative in the United States

What have been the obstacles to the global Baby-Friendly Hospital Initiative in the United States? According to Diony Young, longtime editor of the journal *Birth*, the Department of Health and Human Services and the Department of Agriculture played a part in slowing down the movement in the United States, quite possibly because of pressure from infant-formula corporations, who knew that their profits would be reduced if there was a significant rise in breastfeeding rates here. Instead of protecting breastfeeding, the government decided to protect the infant-formula companies. The American Hospital Association (AHA) has also proved to be an obstacle; in the 1990s it opposed the global initiative as an "unwelcome intrusion and potential expense for hospitals."[30] The pressure from the AHA resulted in proposals to change the definitions and requirements for attaining Baby-Friendly status.

U.S. hospitals face certain obstacles that hospitals in other countries may not in attaining Baby-Friendly certification. Twenty-four-hour rooming-in leaves little reason to maintain large, empty central nurseries. At the same time, there are laws in almost half of the states mandating that every hospital that provides maternity services must maintain a central nursery. This means that the room cannot be converted to a sitting or dining room. One large problem for nurses or pediatricians who would like to see their hospitals become Baby-Friendly is that they have to gain the cooperation of the hospital administrators, obstetricians, midwives, family physicians, postpartum nurses, neonatal intensive-care staff, prenatal services, nutritional services, supplemental food programs, and neighborhood health centers to make it happen. Gaining this cooperation can be hard to achieve when there is still the perception that women don't care whether they breastfeed or not or that the hospital can't do without the free infant formula, luncheons, notepads, pens, pacifiers, newsletters, crib cards, measuring tapes, in-service funds, conference sponsorships, and patient-education materials provided by infant-formula manufacturers.

Baby-Friendly hospitals must also make sure that pregnant and post-partum women are not exposed while in the hospital or its associated clinics to advertising, booklets, calendars, videotapes, or other materials that can undermine breastfeeding and make artificial feeding appear to be the norm. And hospital administrators and staff must make sure that mothers in their care do not leave the hospital with sample products that have been supplied by infant-formula companies to promote their wares. These include discharge gift packs of formula, feeding bottles, nipples, and pacifiers.

Though the U.S. government does enunciate public-health goals (one of which is to achieve a seventy-five percent rate of exclusive breastfeeding by 2010), it can be argued that, compared with the many other countries in the world with higher breastfeeding rates, it does little beyond that to make breastfeeding more attractive, easier, and more possible for our mothers. I would like to see our government put forth a greater effort to increase the number of Baby-Friendly hospitals in this country.

4

GETTING STARTED: THE BASICS

How will you feel immediately after giving birth? You'll know for sure only when that moment arrives. But however your baby's birth happens, there is a very good chance that, besides feeling relieved and elated, you'll be physically exhausted and all of the muscles of your body will want to relax. If so, this is exactly what you should do. Ideally, those who are assisting you will help you find a position in which you don't have to hold any muscle in your body tense.

There is no single perfect position for you to be in to hold your baby for the first time. If you feel strong, it's fine to hold him while seated, but if you feel shaky and exhausted, he can make very nice contact with you if placed facedown on your belly or chest. In fact, if he's breathing well, the best place for him to be is on your belly (or chest), covered with a warm blanket or towel.

Remember: The more uninterrupted skin-to-skin contact you and your baby have during the first two hours after birth, the greater the chance that he will be able to find your breast and latch on to it in the way nature intended. If the hospital where you give birth wants you to wear an open-back hospital gown, I suggest that you turn it around in the latter hour or two of labor so that it opens in the front instead. That way, when your baby is born, he can immediately be placed on your warm, soft skin instead of on the crinkly, uncomfortable sterile paper that is used to cover the examination surfaces in most hospitals. Even if you've had a cesarean, your baby can be placed on your chest for a while if you're feeling well enough. You've done your hard work. Now you're supposed to get comfortable so that you can fully enjoy the precious beginning moments of his life.

Even though your hospital may allow several of your family members in your room soon after you give birth, I recommend that you educate your family that it's better for them to express their love by tidying your house, doing laundry, and preparing meals. The presence of too many loving people around a newborn can overwhelm his senses and cause him to shut down, interfering with his ability to find the breast and learn to suck effectively. Getting a good start to breastfeeding should take priority over getting early photographs. Your baby will appreciate this consideration at the time and probably later in life as well.

When you first hold your baby, he will be wet with amniotic fluid and perhaps some blood if you had a laceration or an episiotomy. He may also have some white cream called vernix on his skin, either in the creases of his arms and legs or, in some cases, all over. If your midwife or nurse wants to wipe away some blood while you are holding your baby, that's okay—although you may prefer to do it yourself. The other fluids are more important, because they are part of nature's signaling system for the next phase of your relationship with your baby to begin. Amniotic fluid and vernix both help to facilitate the process of bonding and attachment. It's as important to let the amniotic fluid and vernix dry on your baby's skin as it is for you to keep soaps and lotions away from your own nipples. Vernix will also protect the skin of your newborn; it will soak in over the next few hours, helping him make the transition between the watery environment he had inside your body and the dry one he'll live in for the rest of his life. If there is a lot of vernix on your baby's back, you'll find what an excellent hand cream it is. Your unwashed baby will exude a wonderful odor, which new mothers often describe in those moments just after birth as "heavenly" or "intoxicating."

Barbara's story shows how much a newborn infant's natural smell can mean to his mother.

Barbara: *Our son was welcomed into our arms after a perfect home birth. The midwife left three hours later, and my husband and I proceeded to call family members with the happy news. My older sister, who lived just an hour away, asked if she could come over to help. She did some laundry, cooked, and then offered to bathe the baby. We didn't think much of it at the time, so I told her to go ahead. I was really surprised after the bath when she handed my baby back to me and I didn't recognize him. I knew it was my baby, but the smell was wrong. This was very upsetting to me. I could never tell my sister this, but this has been one of my most vivid memories of that birth.*

Will you feel an impulse to nuzzle, kiss, or lick your newborn baby? I hope so, and if you do, I invite you to surrender to it. Touch of this kind is calming to a newborn. Your baby will be comforted by your smell, your warmth, and the softness of your breast, even though he may not yet show signs of readiness to suck.

Usually, babies do some licking and nuzzling before getting down to the business of opening their mouths wide enough to really suckle, and

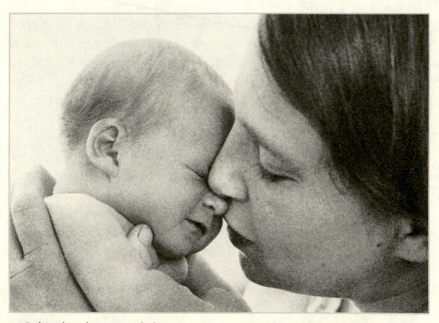

Babies love being nuzzled.

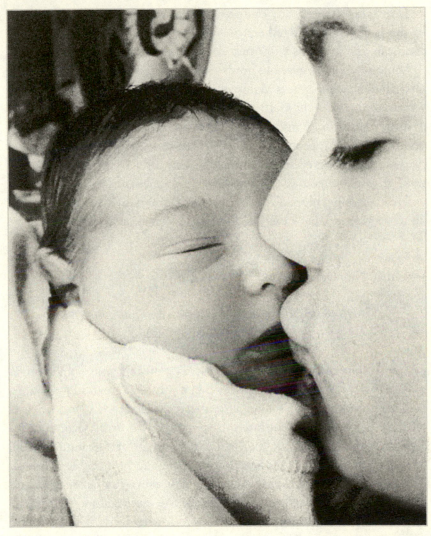

Babies love being kissed.

they're not even ready for the licking and nuzzling until they're breathing freely and easily and feeling somewhat calm. It's always best not to try to force things but rather to let your baby's natural responses unfold in their own time. Pay attention to his movements and signals, as well as to your own sensations and impulses, without hurrying him or becoming upset with your lack of progress. Being in a rush will only make latching more difficult.

Don't think there is any one posture that you should take in order to be doing it "right." Together, you and your baby will find out which positions and practices work best so he gets off to a good start.

Some newborns figure out how to get a good latch at the breast almost immediately, while others require much more time and patience to learn how to feed effectively. Getting a good latch means that your baby is able to draw colostrum or milk from your breast efficiently without injuring your nipples in the process. It may be easier to accomplish this after your placenta has delivered and any stitches you need have been made. Anything that makes you uneasy will have a ripple effect on your baby and will make nursing more difficult. You were your baby's environment for nine months, and that situation does not change once he is born.

Intrinsic Newborn Reflexes and Responses

> *Research findings now support common sense.*
> —Suzanne Colson, PhD

Did you know that your baby's nervous system and your own are programmed to mesh together after birth in a way that creates interactions between the two of you—interactions that can greatly facilitate breast-feeding? Some of the most interesting research on breastfeeding in recent years is the work on "biological nurturing" by Suzanne Colson, PhD, a midwife–researcher based in England and France. Her message is that breastfeeding generally gets off to the best start when mother and baby are able to interact with each other in the ways that mothers themselves find most comfortable in the days following birth. In basic terms, "biological nurturing" is "doing what comes naturally." Although this approach sounds simple and reasonable, it may not be followed in hospitals, where it is common for a new mother to be strongly directed in how to position herself when first introducing her newborn baby to the breast.

Dr. Colson's biological-nurturing approach assumes that both mothers and babies—if they are able to spend uninterrupted time in body contact with each other—exhibit certain behaviors that are intrinsic and instinctual. These very reflexes facilitate effective breastfeeding. Keeping the baby belly-to-belly with the mother often begins the breastfeeding process. Dr. Colson's research suggests that your urges to handle your newborn baby's feet or to give him other kinds of caresses are all part of a familiar pattern of behaviors that trigger your baby's intrinsic responses in preparation for breastfeeding. It's good for you to be able to recognize his cues for what they are, instead of thinking, as overwhelmed new mothers sometimes do, that some of them mean the baby is refusing to take the breast. If your baby turns his head from side to side, this doesn't mean that he is refusing your breast. On the contrary, it means that he is looking for it. More than fifty of these cues have been identified in newborns, including: nuzzling, licking the lips, tongue-darting, snuffling and snorting, opening the mouth, hand to mouth, and bobbing the head.

Your baby is most likely to exhibit these behaviors while next to

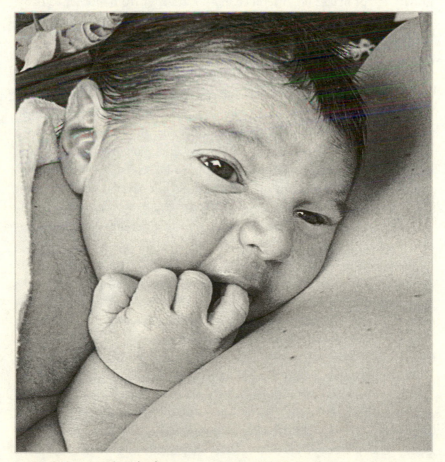

This baby is ready to latch.

your body, especially when he is cuddled up close to you or when you are hugging him. They are clues that he is searching for your breast.

By carefully analyzing videos of feeding sessions of forty healthy mother–baby pairs from England and France during the first month of breastfeeding, Dr. Colson's team found that most of the mothers whose babies exhibited the highest number of inborn reflexes were in a semi-reclined position, with their babies facing toward them in full body contact.[1] This is interesting since, in much breastfeeding literature, this position either isn't mentioned at all or is labeled "incorrect." The current teaching on the subject holds that babies are meant to lie on their backs or sides while feeding and that pressure along the baby's back is necessary for effective feeding. (Maybe people have trouble understanding that the gravity factor makes no difference in milk transfer from mother to baby. No one can drink "uphill" from a cup, but drinking from a breast is another matter.) In the U.K., it is common for a new mother to be instructed that she must sit in an upright position with at least one foot on the floor or lying on her side for there to be a good latch.

Dr. Colson's studies appear to contradict these beliefs, suggesting instead that the positions many mothers take without direction—even nontraditional positions—may be the ones that best trigger the inborn reflexes that help newborns initiate enjoyable, pain-free breastfeeding and satisfactory milk transfer. According to Dr. Colson, "When mothers encountering problems changed to full [biological-nurturing] postures, gulping and gagging diminished, and the baby often became the active agent controlling the feed, aided by the different types of [primitive neonatal reflexes]."

It's worth knowing that one hundred percent of the mothers in the group Dr. Colson's team studied were still breastfeeding at six weeks postpartum (regardless of what position they used for nursing). Compare this with the sixty-three percent in the general U.K. population who were still breastfeeding at this stage after having followed conventional advice from the beginning of their breastfeeding experiences.

When my partners and I began helping mothers initiate breastfeeding during my early days as a midwife, we took the approach that Dr. Colson suggests (although I didn't know her then and she hadn't yet begun her research). We followed the lead of the mother and baby as they moved together. If a mother needed help or encouragement, we gave it. Otherwise, we let nature take its course: We placed the baby on the mother's body

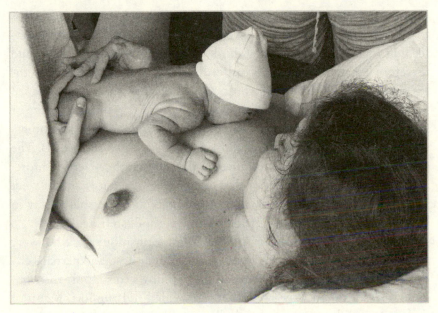

Biological-nurturing position

(making her as comfortable as we could while waiting for the placenta) and let the two of them figure it out for themselves. Very often—but not always—breastfeeding began with the baby still in that position. For each of my own three home births, I chose to lean back with my babies held on top of me. Any other posture would have been less comfortable, from my perspective, just after giving birth. Each of my babies latched perfectly and within half an hour of being born.

In short, Dr. Colson's research buttresses the approach that my partners and I have taken for four decades. Our degree of success in initiating and sustaining breastfeeding is as compelling as it gets (ninety-nine percent initiation of breastfeeding and ninety-seven percent still breastfeeding at six months). We managed this high degree of breastfeeding success without professional advice or manuals, not because we would have rejected either—we just didn't know in our pioneering days that these existed.

Naturally, a semireclined position will not be comfortable for a woman who has just had a cesarean, and not every baby will latch best in the semireclined or fully reclined position. The important consideration is that Dr. Colson observed mothers as they behave of their own accord, without outside interference.

An unexpected observation of one of Dr. Colson's earlier studies was that biological nurturing also increased the length of exclusive breast-feeding for a group of babies who had been considered "at risk" and therefore less likely to enjoy breastfeeding success.[2-3] Some of the mothers involved in these studies chose to sit upright, while others leaned back while sitting, and still others nursed while lying on their backs or sides. Some had complete skin-to-skin contact with their babies; others were lightly clothed (while still allowing easy access to the breast). The mothers who adopted these postures remarked that they were comfortable, with no neck strain and with their shoulders held low and relaxed. Each had good support to all areas of her body and was able to stay in that posture for quite a long period of time without shifting.

Those mothers who were in semireclined positions or who were lying flat on their backs with a pillow under their head and perhaps another under the knees rarely needed more pillows to support their babies. Instead, the mother's own body provided full support. Many of the mothers didn't use their hands for support but instead for caressing and stroking the baby while breastfeeding. In case you've read elsewhere that babies can't get hold of the nipple from this position, this may be true of some tiny premature babies, but most others are fully able to find their mother's nipple and latch on from this position, just as puppies, kittens, and most other mammals do. Newborn babies can scoot forward if placed on their bellies. If they're on their backs, they need to be cuddled so they are lying on one side as they come to the breast.

Babies who are routinely placed on their mothers' abdomen just after birth usually find the breast and latch (with a little help) within an hour. It's best to allow the baby who latches well to stay at the breast until he lets go or falls asleep rather than to interrupt this precious connection because of some external schedule. When your baby is well latched, he has a sense of connection to you and will be able to relax fully. His innate responses function best when he is in this state of mind.

In Dr. Colson's study, some mothers wanted to hold their breasts during a feeding, while others didn't. She concluded that mothers themselves were the best at deciding whether or not to hold the breast and that routine directions (however well meant) about holding the breast can often inhibit mothers' instinctual behaviors. Some women even varied in breast-holding during a feeding from time to time.

Feeding Postures

As you can see, there is no one correct way to hold a feeding baby. Different ways will work better for different women and babies, depending upon the mother's arm length; the size, shape, and height of her breasts; and the baby's mouth habits. It's a good idea to try more than one way if you experience any problems at all in getting started, as you may not yet have discovered what works best for you and your newborn. In these first moments, much will depend upon how your bottom feels right after giving birth and on how tired you are when you first hold your baby.

The Lying Position

If you feel like leaning back with your legs outstretched or with your legs slightly bent at the knees and supported by a pillow, with your feet resting on the bed, go ahead. If your baby is placed immediately on top of you after birth, you are in biological-nurturing position. Not only that—you are also multitasking. Your baby begins to exhibit his inborn reflexes by crawling toward your breasts or massaging them, and your uterus will respond by contracting and expelling your placenta in good time. Bravo! If your bottom is quite sore in the day or so following birth, this semireclining position is likely to work better and be less tiring for you than trying to sit completely upright. It may even allow you to have one or both of your hands free to caress your baby.

The Sitting Position

If you decide that you would be comfortable sitting more upright, you'll probably want a pillow behind your back. You should have two more pillows ready: one for your lap and one for the elbow of the arm holding your baby. A relatively small percentage of women will find that they do not need any pillows, but you should be sure to use one if you must lean forward in order to make contact with his mouth (a forward-leaning posture will cause muscle strain, tension, and backache). Some high-breasted women may find it necessary to prop their baby with more than one pillow. However many pillows you decide to use, be sure to adjust yourself so that there is no strain in your neck and shoulders as you sit, and take a few long, deep breaths as you get settled.

Side-Lying Position

You can also lie on your side with a pillow under your head, holding your baby facing you and in contact with your body. You'll probably want a pillow behind your back as well, because it is important for you to refrain from leaning toward your baby; you should instead be pulling your baby close to you. You may want yet another pillow under your upper leg to achieve a good level of relaxation.

Take note of your baby's position in relation to you before you bring him to your breast. He should be facing you, lying on his side, with his head aligned with the rest of his body. His head should not be tipped way forward or way backward, as this will make swallowing difficult

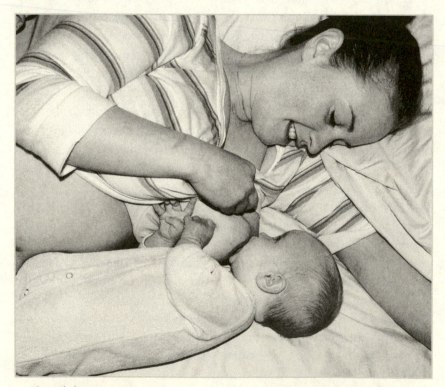

The side-lying position

for him. It is no simpler for babies to swallow this way than it is for adults! Your baby's best nursing position is with his head tilted *slightly* back with his chin gently buried in the underside of your breast.

Always correct your baby's position when you notice that his chin is resting on his chest while nursing. This will not only make it hard for him to swallow, it will soon make your nipples sore. Without detaching your baby, you can simply slide his body about an inch in the direction of his feet. Don't be surprised in the beginning if you have to adjust and readjust your baby in relation to your body until you find what works best for you.

Will your baby's head rest on the bed or on your upper arm as you lie on your side? This depends upon the shape and size of your breasts. As always, choose the posture that is most comfortable for you, adjusting your baby's position accordingly. Once the positioning seems right, you can watch for his "I'm ready" cues (lip-smacking, tongue movements, hands brought to the mouth, or, best, a widely gaped mouth) and, before a moment is lost, pull him toward your breast, aiming so that his chin, not his nose, first contacts your breast. The perfect wide gape, combined with a close cuddle, should result in your baby holding your nipple and areola slightly off center, with a little more of the underside of your breast held firmly in his mouth and his lips flanged outward (someone else might need to look at his lower lip). His body should be tucked in close to yours.

The side-lying position is particularly good for mothers who have had cesareans, as it puts no pressure on the incision, while allowing them to rest comfortably.

Different Ways to Hold Your Baby If Those Already Mentioned Don't Make the Grade

Cradle Hold

As always, step one is to get comfortable. Put a pillow behind your back and shoulders, another under the elbow of the arm that is holding your baby, and—if necessary—another one (sometimes two) in your lap under the baby. It's important that your arms, upper back, and neck do not have to work to support the weight of your baby.

Make sure that he is held snugly to your chest, with his head resting on your forearm, not in the crook of your elbow, and the rest of his body positioned along your arm. He should be lying on his side, with his tummy facing yours and his entire body pulled in close. His lower arm should be tucked under your breast, with his upper arm and hand

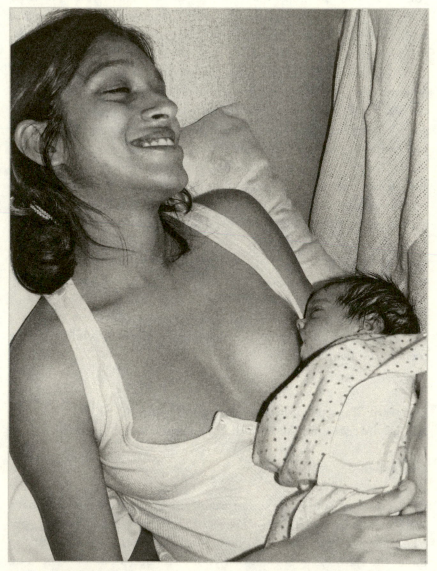

The cradle hold

being held away from his mouth as you bring him toward your breast. His head should be facing straight forward and tilted back just a little, allowing his chin to approach your breast first. If his nose reaches the breast first, a poor latch will be the likely result. If this happens, slide his entire body a little in the direction needed to correct his head position. This move will protect your nipple from an uncomfortable latch at the same time that it will make swallowing much easier for your baby.

Underarm Hold

This feeding position also requires that you get comfortably seated first, with pillows behind your back and shoulders. Arrange one or two at your side to bring your baby up to the level of your breast and then place him on top of these pillows.

Supporting your baby's upper body with your forearm and his neck with your hand, hold him facing you, with the lower half of his body tucked under your arm. You'll want to make sure that his body is positioned so your breast is directly in front of his mouth; he shouldn't have to bend his neck forward in order to latch. Neither you nor your baby should be leaning forward.

When using the underarm hold, it's important that you hold your baby by the back of the neck rather than by the head. In this way, his head is supported, but he is still able to turn it from side to side. Babies don't like having their heads shoved into their food any more than we grown-ups do, and they will resist this if you try it.

Once your baby latches from this position, you can settle back as much as you need to get comfortable. If your arm tires from holding him, you'll need to add another pillow or folded blanket to provide support. (It's possible to develop carpal tunnel syndrome if you make a habit of nursing in this position for weeks without proper support. If you already have carpal tunnel syndrome, you may not like this position.)

The underarm hold may be easier than other positions for women with very large breasts, because it allows a clearer view of the baby while giving the mother better control of the baby's head. It also works well for many women who have had cesareans, because it puts no pressure on the incision. Premature babies with a weak suck may also nurse better in this position.

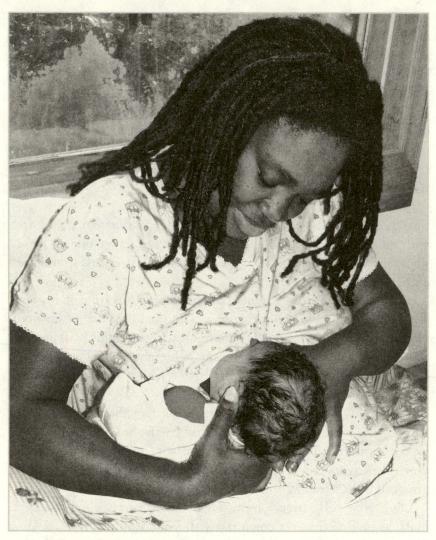

The underarm hold

Cross-Cradle Hold

This seated position is sometimes used for babies who are having a hard time latching (or staying latched) when they are held in a different way. It has sometimes been heavily promoted as the best nursing position, but, in my opinion, it is not a very natural hold—only rarely would a mother discover it on her own. In Australia, I met a few women who continued to use it even though they were having trouble with sore nipples and poor milk transfer. They were simply obeying advice they received just after birth that this position was superior to others, whether or not it was natural-feeling for the mother. Continuing to use this hold once a baby is well latched and breastfeeding may increase your risk of backache and carpal tunnel pain.

Though the cross-cradle hold may involve some difficulties if it becomes the "position of choice," you may find it useful for getting your baby to take your breast for the first few times. Some lactation consultants particularly recommend it for small premature babies, who may still hold themselves in the fetal position while in the cradle hold, thus interfering with a good strong latch.

To use this hold, sit in a comfortable position with enough support behind you so that you are neither leaning back nor forward. Then hold your baby with the arm opposite to the breast you will be offering—in other words, support your baby with your right arm if you want him at your left breast. You will probably need a pillow in your lap to bring your baby up high enough to reach your breast and to support some of his weight. Your baby-holding hand should be supporting your baby's head with your thumb behind his upper ear and your other fingers holding his cheek near his lower ear. Do not push on the back of his head with your hand, as this usually causes babies to arch their backs and to resist. Your other hand (the one on your breast-using side) should cup and support your breast from below. It should be held in a U-shape, with your fingers forming one side of the U, your thumb the other side, and your palm facing upward. Your hand should be below your areola, so that you are sure it is not covering the part of your breast that needs to be inside your baby's mouth.

As with the other feeding positions, you should pull your baby to your breast with his body positioned so that his chin touches your breast first, enabling him to make the ideal off-center latch that protects your nipple from injury and makes it possible for your nipple to be drawn well back into his mouth.

Once your baby is latched well, you can switch from the cross-cradle hold to the cradle hold, which you will probably find more relaxing.

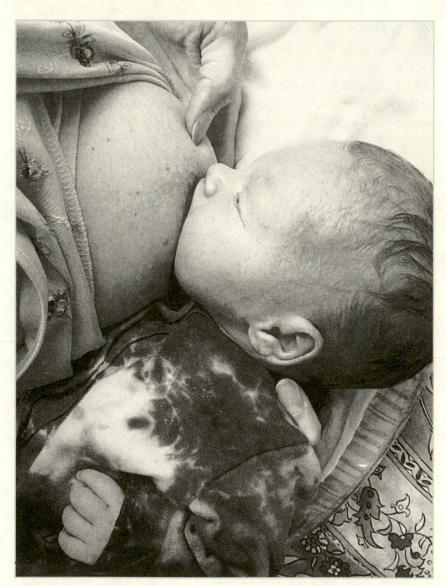

The cross-cradle hold

Other Positions

There are a few more acrobatic positions that may prove temporarily useful if you are having problems with injured nipples or an obstructed milk duct. If the obstructed duct is above your areola, for instance, you might find it useful to nurse your baby with his feet held toward your head. Or you might lay your baby on his back as you crouch over him on your elbows and knees in order to find the alignment between his body and yours that puts his chin on the place closest to your blocked duct.

To Hold or Not to Hold Your Breast

The advantage of holding your breast when you and your baby are learning effective feeding is that proper holding can make your breast firmer, which will make latching on easier for your baby. Your holding hand becomes a one-cup living bra. However, it's important to hold your breast correctly if you don't want to introduce secondary problems. Whether you use the C-hold or the U-hold, your hand needs to be positioned well back from the areola. Check this carefully, and make sure that you are presenting your baby with a nipple that is being squeezed into a shape that can fit into his mouth (an oval that's lying down).

If your breasts are rather small, holding your breast with one hand may not be necessary at all.

Sometimes women with really large breasts find it easier to put a pillow under the breast to support its bulk, using one hand to support the part near (close to, but never over) the areola.

Once your baby has become an adept eater, you'll probably find that he has no trouble maintaining a good latch without your hand supporting the weight of your breast. However, as long as he sometimes loses hold of a good latch when he'd rather be suckling, it's a good idea to continue holding your breast while nursing. It won't be long until he's strong enough to keep his grasp with less help.

It will be easier for your crying baby to latch well if you calm him before bringing him to your breast.

Knowing If the Latch Is Right

To qualify as a correct latch to the breast (rather than a signal that you need to protect your nipple and try again), the latch should have your baby's lips curled outward and firmly applied to your breast. If your breasts are large, you will find it hard to see for yourself, but this is what should be happening if your baby has a good latch: If you pull slightly on your baby's lower lip while he is suckling, you should see that his tongue is curled up on each side and cupped around your breast, form-

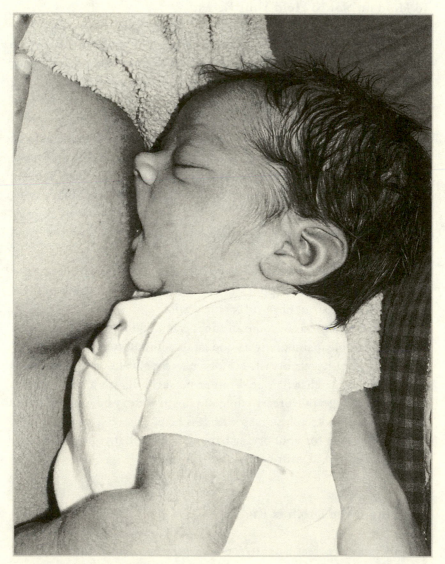

A good latch

ing a trough to the back of his mouth. A large area of his tongue should be in direct contact with the underside of your breast, massaging it in a wavelike motion that brings the milk into his mouth with every suck.

Other Signs of a Good Latch:

- You hear your baby swallowing—*gulp, gulp, gulp.*

- You can see movement at the place between your baby's temple and ear.

- You hear no clicking or smacking sound as your baby sucks (indicating that he is breaking and reestablishing suction again and again).

- Your breast is greatly softened after the baby feeds there.

- Your nipple doesn't hurt after the first few sucks.

- Your baby seems relaxed when he's feeding.

Signs of a Bad Latch

When your baby is nursing, there should be absolutely no friction taking place between the baby's mouth and your breast, and your breast should not be pulled in and out as he sucks. If you or someone else sees this happening, it's time to end this incorrect latch and start again, even if you have to repeat the process thirty-seven times. Remember, you are not a failure as a mother if your baby decides that it is too much trouble to nurse and goes to sleep before achieving a good latch. Soon enough, he will wake up again, wanting to suck. If you are patient and persistent, newborn babies can learn new habits fairly quickly, because, unlike adults, they live completely in the present moment and do not cling to the past or worry about the future. One thing to remember, though, is that it will be easier for you to teach your baby to correct his latch if your immediate surroundings are not full of distractions.

Another sure sign that your baby's latch needs correction is when your nipple has been sucked into an asymmetrical shape just after nursing. For example, you may notice that it has been drawn into the shape of a new lipstick.

Fixing Your Baby's Latch

If your baby has trouble latching, it may be that you are leaning forward and trying to aim your breast dead center into your baby's mouth. This strategy is likely to make your baby grasp your nipple only in the front part of his mouth, which will be bad news for your nipple. I like the sandwich analogy, as described by Diane Wiessinger, a U.S. lactation consultant and La Leche League leader. She points out that when you are going to take a bite out of a large sandwich, your lower jaw is the movable part and, in taking that first bite, you will position it well back into the underside of the sandwich. Your upper jaw will be the last part to complete the bite. Think of this approach as you bring your baby's mouth to your breast. Instead of making a bull's-eye approach—trying to get your nipple centered in your baby's mouth—try instead to have his head tilted slightly back so his chin reaches your breast before his mouth. Pull him toward you so that your breast is rolled onto his lower jaw first; this way, he can take a large mouthful of the underside of your areola. Your areola should go into his mouth a split second before your nipple gets there. Just as your nipple begins to disappear into his mouth and his jaws start to close, pull his shoulders in even closer to your body. Doing this gives him a better chance of getting your nipple (and much of your areola) well back into his mouth.

Wait to bring your baby toward your breast until his mouth is about as wide as a yawn. Think of how baby birds ask for food from their parents. If your baby doesn't open wide, there are a few strategies for encouraging better gaping. One is to gently tickle and tease his lips with your nipple. Another is to hold your own mouth open wide. (Researchers have demonstrated what countless mothers already knew: Newborn babies come equipped with the ability to imitate facial expressions.) Another is to press your baby's palm. If all these methods fail to produce the response you want, you can gently and firmly pull down on his chin with the index finger of the hand that is supporting your breast. Do this only as your baby is opening his mouth—the act of opening puts his mind into a relaxed state, so you shouldn't encounter resistance at that moment. It may help you to obtain assistance if you have trouble coordinating all the movements necessary to accomplish this. Timing is everything, and practice makes perfect.

Getting Baby to Let Go

Knowing how to get your baby to let go of your breast once he has latched on incorrectly is an indispensable skill. I have noticed that many women will put up with nipple pain rather than end a bad latch in order to try again—as if they are afraid to disturb the baby once he is sucking, even if he isn't well latched and it hurts. The trouble with this is that nipple tissue can easily be injured, and when this happens, that injury can quickly worsen, inhibiting your baby's ability to get your milk. Remember: When the latch is bad, he isn't getting much milk, so please don't be afraid to stop an unsatisfactory latch until he gets it right. There are several methods that you might use:

- Push down on your breast near the corner of your baby's mouth and quickly pull your nipple out.

- Put your finger into the corner of his mouth to break suction.

- Pull down on his chin.

Don't be surprised if you have to make your baby let go many times as you learn together how to get the latch right. Neither you nor he will be graded on your performance. He is depending upon you to teach him how to get eating right. Once this skill is learned, he will remember how to do it, because the reward will be great.

The most important thing is that your baby must attach to you in a way that doesn't hurt you. If it is a real stretch for you to say that the first latch feels comfortable and good, you should break the suction between his lower lip and your breast by pushing down on your breast at the corner of his mouth, then deftly and quickly snatch your nipple out of reach of his gums. Most babies will be surprised but not upset or angry if you do this.

Remember that you need to be attentive to your nipples' sensitivity right from the beginning. You are not supposed to tolerate your little one gumming your nipples, so don't tell yourself that you can probably stand it or that you are undergoing something that is normal. Your nipples are not supposed to "toughen up" or become blistered, red, raw, or shaped asymmetrically after your baby has been suckling. Your baby can and must learn how to latch on correctly. However, this learning takes place only when you go through the routine of disconnecting and then reintroducing the breast, trying for a better latch. Mother animals in the wild instinctively make sure that their little ones get sucking right rather than putting up with unnecessary pain. With them, suckling is about feeling good as much as it is about making sure their young ones thrive.

There is no reason to put a time limit on how long your baby feeds from each breast. It's actually a good idea to let him decide when to let go of one side before you offer the other, because this allows him to get both the thirst-quenching foremilk and the higher-calorie hindmilk.

5

YOUR BABY'S NEEDS—AND YOURS—
DURING THE FIRST WEEK

Healthy full-term babies whose mothers have received little or no medication are almost always born wide awake and aware. They prefer rather dim lights to bright ones and their mother's arms to anyone else's. Like other newborn mammals, they come equipped with an awareness of their own vulnerability, and they don't want to be alone. Having spent the entire pregnancy within your body, your baby is going to be comforted by the relaxed loving presence of the most familiar person in the world—you (or her father). She will feel best when she's being held by you, but she will enjoy being held by another person who loves her if you are not able to hold her right away.

After two or three hours in this state of quiet alertness—characterized by bright, wide-open eyes—your baby may begin to show signs of drowsiness and drift off to sleep. In fact, most of her first forty-eight hours will be spent asleep. Three- to four-hour naps are common on the first two days, punctuated by relatively short periods of alert wakefulness.

A small amount of colostrum will satisfy your healthy full-term baby's need for liquid for the first two days, so there is no need for her to be given extra nourishment. In fact, giving newborns sugar water at this time can interfere with the initiation of breastfeeding by filling your baby's tiny stomach, thus taking away her motivation to suckle. She then gets less colostrum and your breasts don't receive the stimulation they need to get your milk production off to a strong start. If your baby is born between 35 and 39 weeks (the definition of late-preterm), she may look mature, but many of these babies are less vigorous suckers and tend to sleep far more than those who are born at term. They have two to four times the risk for respiratory distress, infection, jaundice, and hospitalization for more than five days. To minimize such risk, it is best to give them supplemental feedings during the first hour or two of life with colostrum you expressed and froze during pregnancy. If your early baby goes right to the breast and is a hearty sucker, this is good. If not, supplement with your colostrum by dropper.

The use of a bottle during the early days of life can interfere with her learning to suck effectively, since the mechanics of receiving milk from an artificial nipple and bottle are so different from drawing milk from your breast. One well-designed study showed that breastfed babies who were given extra water or formula during the first few days actually lost *more* weight and were slower to start gaining by the fourth day than babies who were exclusively breastfed or formula-fed.[1] Late-preterm babies, on the other hand, don't have these energy reserves. They need early colostrum, as much skin-to-skin contact as possible, and careful assessment of their ability to get your milk. Remember: Some babies appear to be sucking, but they may not be swallowing. If you aren't sure your baby is actually swallowing, ask the nurse to listen to her throat with a stethoscope as she nurses.

If you have diabetes, then your baby is at risk for hypoglycemia (low blood sugar). It is important that she gets colostrum within the first hour after birth, whether directly from the breast or by supplementation with your expressed colostrum. Over the next three to four hours, nurse or supplement once each hour. Over the next eight hours, try to nurse every two to three hours.

If you are diabetic or obese, it will take longer for your milk to come in, so you should begin to either hand-express or pump right away, as this will reduce any delay in milk production.

Many Babies Aren't Born Hungry

As previously mentioned, newborn babies almost always lose some weight during the first three to four days of life, whether they are nursed or artificially fed. This is normal. The majority of this weight loss is due to the expulsion of meconium, the odorless substance inside your baby's intestines during pregnancy that keeps them from sticking together as they develop. When she is born and begins to drink colostrum, a natural laxative, the meconium is expelled; it may weigh as much as half a pound (227 g). Your baby's weight loss may also be partly from normal fluid loss.

Since most people aren't aware that a five- to seven-percent loss of a healthy full-term baby's birth weight is normal during the first days of life, one of the biggest surprises of the first two days is that—though they will want to suck—many babies aren't born hungry. Nature prepares newborns for birth by filling the liver and other vital organs with enough nutrition in the form of glycogen to sustain the baby for two or three days. True hunger usually arrives on day three or four, around the time that milk production ordinarily begins. Newborn behavior may vary, though, according to how much medication the baby received from drugs given to the mother during labor.

This observation is worth remembering if you have one of those babies who don't appear to be hungry for the first two days. When mothers get worried about their babies losing weight just after birth, I usually remind them of the 1985 earthquake that struck Mexico City. I remember a report from the rescuers, who, ten days after the earthquake, were still pulling victims from the rubble at the site of a ten-story hospital. During the first week of rescue work, adult survivors were sometimes found alive, but after ten days, the only survivors found were several newborn babies—they were the only humans who had the energy stores to live for such a long time without a drop to eat or drink.

When to Offer Your Breast

Offer your breast to your baby whenever she is in a quiet alert state during the first two days. If she is crying or fussy, relax yourself by breathing slowly and deeply, and calm her by holding her near your breast. These beginning moments together are irreplaceable, and you'll find that your memories of this time will persist throughout your life, so it's worth making them as special as they can be.

Don't take it as rejection if your baby doesn't spend a lot of time suckling during the first two days of life. Some babies will take the breast only once or twice on the first day but will become more eager to latch on the second or third day. The baby who was such a quiet soul on the first day often shows everyone how many decibels she can reach during the following two. This can be alarming the first time it happens, since the behavior is different from what you've seen before. Learn to take a deep, deep breath if you find that your baby's cry causes you to clench any of your muscles. Do what you feel like to comfort her, whether it's holding her close, talking to her, or singing to her. These behaviors should help both of you relax.

The Appearance of Colostrum and Milk

Colostrum ranges in color from clear to creamy yellow. Your milk, though, ranges from bluish-white (foremilk) to a whiter color (hindmilk). Sometimes milk turns blue, green, or pink, depending upon what you've been eating (food colorings and some foods can affect the color of your milk without harming it).

How to Know That You Are Meeting Your Baby's Needs

Once your milk comes in, the best way to tell how your baby is doing is to count the number of wet or poopy diapers she gives you. Those babies who are breastfed exclusively don't pee often during the first day of life; in fact, most pee just once by the end of the first day (some pee as they are being born, but this may not be noted). Most babies make two wet diapers by day two and three on day three of life. It is easier for an inexperienced person to detect a wet diaper if the diaper is cloth rather than an ultra-absorbent disposable diaper, which doesn't feel wet when it is.

Once your milk begins to come in—usually on day three, four, or five—the number of wet diapers per day will increase dramatically. By the end of the first week, you can tell that your baby is getting enough fluids if she gives you six to eight soaking wet cloth diapers (five or six disposable diapers) within a twenty-four-hour period.

Poop is different. Your baby should poop within twenty-four hours of being born, and she is likely to have several meconium poops during the first two days of life. Meconium is black or greenish-black and sticky, so on days one and two her poop will be like this as well. On days three and four, it will turn several shades lighter and be less sticky as her body expels the remaining meconium and she starts to drink milk. By day four or five, a breastfed baby's poop will turn yellow, and will no longer be sticky and odorless, because all the meconium will have been expelled. You should be getting three to four of these poopy diapers within a twenty-four-hour period (to count as a poopy diaper, the stained area should be as large as a large grape). Sometimes the poop has an irregular consistency and is curdy, and at other times it can be watery. Regardless of the consistency, it's almost always yellow. (A grandmother used to formula-fed babies might be surprised at the yellow color, since formula-fed baby poop is usually green, harder than breast-milk poop, and smellier.) If your baby's poop is still dark and watery by day five and she hasn't started to gain weight, it may be that you are switching from one breast to the other too soon, causing her to miss out on the more calorie-rich hindmilk. Seek the advice of your knowledgeable lactation consultant or pediatrician.

Besides these signs, you can tell if your baby is suckling well and getting enough milk if:

- There are all the signs of a good latch (see page 97).

- There is movement just in front of your baby's ears while she is sucking.

- Nursing feels good to you.

- When your baby is finished (after ten to twenty minutes), she lets go of your breast.

Your letdown reflex should also be working well. One way to tell is to pay attention to whether your other breast drips or sprays when your baby suckles on one side. You may even find yourself leaking when the usual time for a feeding approaches. (The letdown reflex does not necessarily cause leaking in everyone.) Most women find that they can stop such leaking by pressing directly on the nipple with a forearm or the heel of one hand, or by gently twisting the nipple. A friend of mine leaked so much during the night during the first six months that she took several towels to bed with her to keep her sheets from getting soaked. On the other hand, some women see dripping or spraying only when they are submerged in warm water or leaning forward. You'll know that your milk is letting down if you experience one or more of the following signs:

- Milk leaking from the other breast.

- Tingling in the breasts, with a feeling of overflowing.

- Uterine cramps.

- Your baby's sucking slows during the feeding.

- You see milk in the corner of your baby's mouth.

- You feel more relaxed.

It's a little more difficult to figure out whether you are meeting your baby's emotional needs, but it will help you to remember that newborn babies live in the present moment. They don't think about their experiences; they just experience. When they're awake, they want to be held or talked to. They want (and will reward) your undivided attention, which means that you need to keep your attention in the present as well. Keeping your attention on your baby is an extremely important way to meet her immediate needs; it will help you learn her cues and eventually be a more confident mother.

Your Baby's Growth

Your breastfed baby should gain about six ounces per week during the first three or four months, and she should grow about one inch per month. If you give birth in a hospital, your baby will be weighed every day during your stay. This doesn't mean that it's *necessary* for her to be weighed on the first two days after the initial exam, as diaper-counting gives better information. My partners and I usually check the baby's weight at the age of one week or ten days. If you weigh her at the age of one week, you should figure the weight gain from the lowest weight that she reached. It will take your breastfed baby an average of five to six months to double her birth weight. If she was born prematurely or ill, you can expect that it may take longer for her to reach the normal weight gain.

Skills to Learn During the First Week

Burping

Once your milk comes in and your baby has a full tummy, knowing how to help your baby burp can be a good thing. The time to try is when she has fed for a while and has released your breast. Sit her upright in your lap, supporting her jaw and chest with one hand and gently rubbing and patting her back with your other. Any bubble that's in her tummy will soon rise to the top. You can also hold her draped over your shoulder with a diaper underneath for protection and pat her back. After a burp, she may want to resume feeding. What if she doesn't burp after you've held her upright for two or three minutes? Don't worry about it.

Don't be surprised if your baby spits up milk now and then during the first week. In fact, with some babies, this may go on for four months or so. Spitting up is normal behavior in young babies, and it usually passes by the time they are able to sit up on their own. Lots of babies spit up every day and continue to gain a healthy amount of weight. You can prevent some instances of spitting up by keeping your baby upright just after a feeding and by refraining from putting pressure on her tummy. Avoid dressing her in baby clothes with tight elastic waistbands.

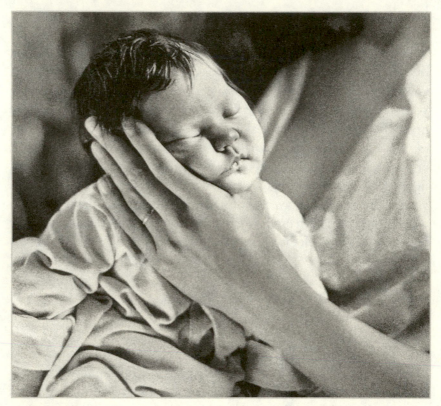

Burp hold

Swaddling

Some babies have trouble taking the breast during the first week or two because they don't realize that they have to move their hands away from their mouths in order to get a good latch. When you try to move one hand away from her mouth, the other instantly takes its place, and you and your baby soon become too frustrated to connect. Don't despair. Cultures all over the world have dealt with this problem by passing down the custom of swaddling to successive generations. Swaddling is a way of wrapping the baby tightly in a blanket to calm her. Young babies are used to being in a confined space (your womb), and many feel insecure when they aren't being held as snugly as they were inside.

Here's the method I find easiest:

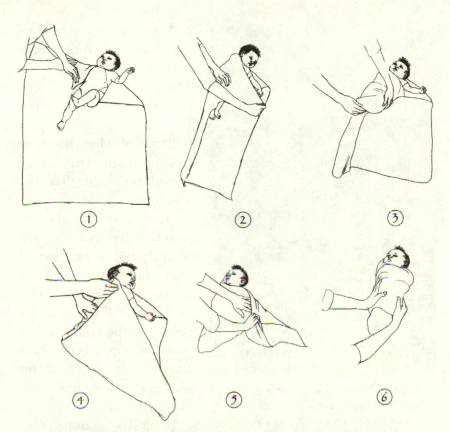

1. Fold one blanket corner down, and lay your baby over that fold. Fold the opposite corner over baby's arm. 2. Bring baby's wrapped arm over his or her chest. 3. Tuck the corner snugly under baby's back. 4. Fold the bottom of the blanket up. 5. Fold the other blanket edge over baby's free arm, and bring that arm over baby's chest. 6. Tuck that corner tightly under baby's back.

I use swaddling mainly to help a jittery or fussy baby take her mother's breast without frustration. Swaddling is not a good idea if your baby is gaining slowly as it prevents the skin-to-skin contact that will help your baby stimulate a greater milk supply.

Hand Expression

One of the skills you will find extremely useful is hand expression of your milk. It's a good idea to learn how to do this before you really need

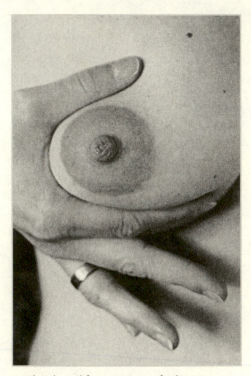

Thumb and finger position for beginning hand expression. Begin with backward motion toward your chest, then roll forward.

it. Many women learn during pregnancy. Your breasts might become overfull when you're away from your baby; manual expression will probably be the quickest way to feel relieved. Hint: It's easier to express milk from your breast before rather than after a feeding.

Hold your breast with your thumb placed an inch to an inch and a half behind your nipple on the upper side of your breast, and your first two fingers (held close together) at the same distance from your nipple below. Your areola isn't a good guide for placement, since women's areolas vary so much in size.

Begin by pressing your thumb and middle finger back toward your chest wall, taking care not to make pressure with your last two fingers on the rest of your breast. Now roll your thumb toward your nipple as if you were making a thumbprint; at the same time, change from middle finger pressure to index finger pressure below. With this motion, you are imitating what your baby's mouth does while sucking. Repeat this rolling motion rhythmically. You may have to repeat the sequence a few times before your milk begins to flow. Be careful not to squeeze or pull on your breast or nipple.

If you have trouble with this technique, you might find that you have better luck if you are in a shower or a warm bath. It may also help if you roll just behind your nipple gently between your thumb and first two fingers before trying to hand-express milk. Stroke your breast from the chest wall toward your nipple a few times.

Once the milk flow slows or stops, you can rotate your fingers forty-five degrees and then ninety degrees and repeat the process so that you express the milk from all sectors of your breast.

It's important to remember that hand expression should not hurt. If it does, you are being too rough with yourself. Once you become adept at hand expression, you may find it possible to express from both breasts at once.

Challenges You May Face in Getting Started

More Than Enough Milk

Some women produce much more milk than their babies can swallow. The baby who chokes and pulls away from the breast just when your milk lets down is doing her best not to drown in too much of a good thing. A baby who has trouble dealing with how fast your milk flows will often do better when you are semireclined or lying flat with her on top of you. Side-lying can be good as well, as it allows milk to dribble out of her mouth instead of running into the back of her throat and forcing her to gulp fast to keep from choking.

Pay attention to your baby's head position while feeding, making sure that it's correct—tilted back slightly with her chin slightly up (not resting on her chest). When her throat is open like this, it is much easier for her to swallow. Allow your baby to pull away whenever she needs to, as you don't want her to feel that she can't come away from the breast when the milk is coming too fast. Since she is most likely getting more than enough of the thirst-quenching but less rich foremilk in her feedings, it may be a good idea to put her to feed at the same breast for three or four consecutive sessions so that she will remove enough of the foremilk to get to the richer hindmilk before moving on to the other breast. Fully emptying one breast before introducing the baby to the other will help signal your body to adjust milk production. Please note: This may not be the best strategy if your baby is gaining less than seven ounces per week. When figuring her weight gain, count from her lowest weight, not from the birth weight.

Burp your baby frequently if she seems to take in air while swallowing fast.

The Baby Who Falls Asleep at the Breast

Some babies will suckle a couple of times and then fall asleep while still latched, particularly in the first few days, when the baby is still logy from being born. To keep your baby awake and actively suckling, it may help to stop the feeding, take off all her clothing except for a diaper, massage her feet, walk your fingers up her spine, or tickle her under her chin or behind her neck. Do this, of course, in a warm room. A baby who is hard for Mom to wake up may do so more easily if Dad is the one who stimulates her to drink more. Babies who fall asleep easily at the breast sometimes stay awake better if you make sure that they are very alert before you begin. As your baby gets older, she will be less likely to fall asleep after a few sucks.

A baby who sips, sleeps, and sips like this quickly wears her mother out. It's best to keep her at the same breast for several feedings, to make sure she's getting your more-filling hindmilk.

How often should you try to wake your baby at your breast? It depends on whether or not she is swallowing. If she needs to gain weight and she tends to go back to sucking and swallowing when awakened, it's a good idea to continue the feeding. You may find that compressing your breast manually to quicken your milk flow will suffice to keep your baby awake and drinking. Learn how to time the compressions to the rhythm of her swallowing. Dr. Jack Newman's website has some excellent clips related to this skill at: http://www.drjackman.com. If you don't succeed immediately in waking your drowsy baby, perhaps you can both take a wonderful nap—you deserve the rest.

Babies Who Refuse the Breast

Some babies refuse the breast during the first few days after birth. There may be several reasons for this behavior, but the important thing to recognize is that the baby may be quite willing to take the breast at a later time. It's good not to give up too easily. Of course, it can be frustrating—even frightening—when your baby doesn't easily latch on to your breast.

Sometimes the problem arises because your baby didn't get to spend uninterrupted time in skin-to-skin contact with you just after birth.

Babies who miss going to the breast during the first hour or two after birth may refuse the breast at first when returned to their mothers' arms and then seem to have little feeling about what to do with it. Or, if your baby had trouble breathing after birth and was given a deep suctioning or intubation, she may be reacting by drawing her attention away from the part of her body that received the greatest insult—the mouth and throat. This reaction can be strong enough to temporarily override the inborn urge to root and suckle. If either of these is a likely cause for why your baby doesn't want to accept your breast, the question then becomes how to encourage her normal responses to return. It is necessary to woo your baby with sweet feelings and associations. A good first step is to nuzzle or kiss your baby and then to manually express some colostrum or milk and get it on her lips or tongue. Above all, don't move quickly or communicate any sense of hurry or urgency. Playfulness and patience are necessary. Talk or sing to your little one, and try to make any time at your breast as pleasant as possible. Calm her before bringing her back to your breast if she becomes upset and starts turning away or arching backward. I know of one father—a farmer—who helped solve his baby's breast refusal by imitating the behavior he had observed in his nanny goats in similar situations. Like the goats, he tried licking his baby, and it worked. The principles that I have just described are applicable to overcoming breast refusal, no matter what the reason for it may be.

If the breast refusal begins at the end of the first week, the problem may stem from breast engorgement, tongue-tie, or a slow letdown—all of which I discuss in greater detail in the next chapter. Other babies may refuse to latch on if they are sleepy and lethargic because they aren't getting enough milk (stimulation of the baby's feet in such a case may encourage her to feed more effectively). It's also possible that your baby is still feeling the effects of any painkilling medications you were given around the time of her birth.

Ordinarily, there is no reason to wake a sleeping baby. However, if your milk supply seems well established and you are near the end of the first week without getting the number of wet or poopy diapers you need per day, waking your sleepy baby may be worth trying. It will be easier to wake her from a light sleep rather than a deep one, so it's a good idea to learn to distinguish between the two states. Signs of light sleep are rapid eye movements beneath the eyelids, arm- and leg-twitching, and changes in facial expression; babies in deep sleep no longer move in these ways.

If you decide to wake your baby for nursing, make sure that the room is dimly lit and that you unwrap her from any blankets. Talk to her and try to get eye contact. A gentle massage of her bare feet is one pleasant wake-up technique, and a diaper change is also a good way of waking her. Once your sleepy baby is awake, plenty of skin-to-skin contact, touch, and massage will encourage her to feed. If she gets sleepy at one breast, you might try using the underarm hold rather than the cuddle hold. If sleepiness and lethargy persist throughout the first week, contact a lactation consultant or peer counselor.

Babies, uncivilized little beings that they are, don't prefer perfume, deodorant, scented lotions, shampoos, or conditioners to the way you happen to smell at any given time. In fact, some babies find these smells so overwhelming (and confusing) that they will not accept the breast when you are wearing a perfumed product. Your baby will love the way you smell even if you happen to be soaked with sweat and spilled milk. This is wonderful, when you think about it.

I have also seen babies refuse the breast during the first two or three weeks because their mothers were taking a DHA supplement that gave their milk a strong, unpleasant taste (not all have an unpleasant taste). Make sure to thoroughly taste any supplements you are taking as well as your own milk to see if this might be a reason for breast refusal.

Babies learn best when they are quickly rewarded for correct behavior. The best reward is your milk, however you can get it into your baby's mouth. Expressing a few drops before you bring her to your breast is often a good way to encourage her to open wide enough to accept your breast well. If your baby doesn't open wide and latch when you draw her to your breast, hold her away from your breast for a few seconds (this is better than continuing to hold her so that her lips are touching it, hoping that she will latch correctly next time, as she's more apt to give up or get mad this way). With a couple of drops on your nipple, draw her to you so that her chin is the first part of her face to touch the underside of your breast. When she gapes wide, hold her close. If she begins suckling, compress your breast with your free hand to start your milk flowing.

If your baby still hasn't latched well after three or four days, you must contact someone who is experienced at helping babies to latch correctly—for example, a lactation consultant, a midwife, or even another nursing mother. In the meantime, you may need to pump milk and give this expressed milk to your baby via syringe or a supplemental nursing system (SNS) to get enough calories into her. Sometimes, a breast shield can solve the problem.

It will encourage you to know that even if your baby gets off to a slow start with nursing, she can still get the hang of it if you are persistent. I know a mother—Esther—whose baby refused the breast for months before finally starting to nurse.

❧ **Esther:** *My first two babies were born at home and nursed easily for many months. My third baby, Eric, was born at home three weeks early. He became jaundiced soon after birth, so my midwife wanted him to be checked by a pediatrician. Off we went to the hospital on his second day of life. The residents who saw him scared me with talk about complete blood transfusion, which turned out not to be necessary. With all of the worry and excitement, Eric never managed to latch on, and he became dehydrated. They did a spinal tap on him to try to find out what was wrong, and he was given antibiotics to cover a possible infection (although they never really diagnosed this as his problem). The antibiotics gave him thrush, and that caused nursing to be hard for both of us. He would occasionally manage to get a few swallows of milk, but he wouldn't stay on very long. It was too much work. He would fuss at me when I would put him to my breast. I would look at him, and he would get yellower as he cried and fussed.*

We kept at this for about a week. Nursing him was painful for me. It was very stressful to keep trying while he cried and fussed and then to pump and teaspoon-feed him or try to feed him my milk from a cup. I got so tired in the shoulders that I would just hurt.

Finally I gave up on breastfeeding, because I would show him my breast and he would start to arch his back and cry. My breast had become an unhappy place. But knowing how good breastfeeding is, I gave myself the short-term goal of pumping my milk for six months, so I could feed him my expressed milk. Fortunately, I was good at manually expressing milk.

When Eric was four and a half months old, he began sucking on his fists and making noises. I thought, if you can put both fists in your mouth, try this. He took it on the first try. That day was relatively easy. I was so happy, because it seemed like a miracle. When I called my lactation consultant, she said, "Don't give him a bottle. Try your hardest, Esther, whatever it takes. Keep offering the breast first." The next day he was medium about it. On the third day, he got mad and cried a lot, but I kept telling him, "This is it. This is how you get your food." I put all the bottles out of sight, and I offered him spoonsful of milk a couple of times. After the third day he quit resisting, and there was no more trouble. His best nursing was at night, when we were both half asleep.

Nipple Shields

Sometimes a baby fails to latch well during the first few days because she never manages to get the breast far enough back into her mouth to trigger effective sucking. The thin, soft silicone shields that are now available can often help a baby like this to get a good latch, because the shield can be long enough to reach the part of her mouth that triggers a good suckling response. The ideal length of the nipple shield would be

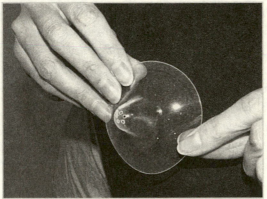

between two and three centimeters. A good fit is important, so if a nipple shield doesn't work for you, the problem may have to do with the size and shape of the shield. If you have trouble getting the shield to stay in place on your breast, it may help to dip it into warm water before applying it.

Nipple shield

Fiona's story shows how valuable nipple shields can be in teaching some babies a good latch.

Fiona: *When Heather was born, I lost a lot of blood. She didn't nurse for the first twenty-four hours or so because I was quite weak. After that, it took longer for my milk to come in. I think it was pretty hard for her, waiting for the milk, because she cried a lot and got very irritated every time I tried to put her to my breast. Also, my nipples tend to be sort of flat, which I think added to her frustrations, as she was having trouble latching on.*

She latched on successfully only a couple of times during the first few days. My mom said that I had similar problems latching when I was born and that she had used a nipple shield for the first few days. I remember feeling reluctant to try one at first because I was afraid that Heather would get attached to it. The shield helped a lot and allowed Heather to nurse well.

I tried a few times without the shield, but it really made her upset, and she was still struggling to latch on without it. After hearing her hungry cry for so many days, I wanted to do whatever made her happy and just let her nurse with the shield. Periodically I'd try nursing without the shield, but she didn't seem interested and I didn't try long.

At around three weeks, I began feeling like I wanted to wean Heather off the shield. I found a forum online where some other women had written about their experience with the shield, and they gave some suggestions of things that had helped in the weaning process.

In the end, it was catching Heather when she was drowsy that did it. She was more willing to try when she was sleepy, and my nipple had been drawn out some at this point, so she had more success latching on. I think it took about a week to wean her completely. She needed the shield less and less until it was just a memory.

Physiologic Jaundice

Good research has shown that babies who breastfeed at least ten times during their first day of life are less likely to develop physiologic jaundice than babies who had fewer feedings. This seems to happen because colostrum has a laxative effect and the excess bilirubin is expelled in the meconium. The baby who gets only a little bit of colostrum will not eliminate the bilirubin so quickly, and this bilirubin can then be reabsorbed into the baby's blood and cause jaundice.

Don't worry, though, if your baby doesn't want to feed ten times on the first day. Many perfectly healthy babies will take two or three days to build up to ten feedings per day, with no negative impact. If they also have signs of physiologic jaundice, it may take a little longer for this jaundice to clear than if the baby was interested in more feedings somewhat earlier.

It's important to know that jaundice occurs in young babies in more than one form. Physiologic (normal) jaundice is the most common kind, and it is quite harmless. This type of jaundice shows up between day two and day five of life and then subsides, causing no problem to the baby. The more immature the baby, the longer it usually takes for this type of jaundice to disappear. Bilirubin, the yellow pigment that characterizes jaundice, is produced in the liver with the breakdown of old or damaged red blood cells. It must then be excreted by the body. Newborn babies' livers are still somewhat immature and therefore take a little while to get rid of this excess bilirubin.

Jaundice is usually considered pathologic (a sign of disease) when it is present in the first two days after birth. When this happens, it's a good idea to have the baby's blood tested. Other signs of jaundice that may be pathologic rather than physiologic are 1) a deepening of the yellow hue of the skin, 2) when jaundice is present in a baby who is born anemic, 3) when there is a pronounced rise in the baby's bilirubin level in the days following birth, and 4) when the baby is lethargic.

No matter whether jaundice in a newborn is physiologic or pathologic, breastfeeding should be continued.

Your Own Needs and Feelings

Your needs will be fairly simple during the first two or three days. You'll be thirsty, hungry, perhaps sore, and you'll need as much rest as you can get. You will need the help of others. Traditionally, women received care from members of their extended family around this time. Family members prepared food, kept the house clean, looked after older children, and provided any necessary advice and encouragement for breastfeeding. If you have no relative or friend who can help you in this way, good planning can help make the first week or two after birth much easier. Get your grocery shopping done before you give birth, and put plenty of easy-to-prepare food in your freezer. If you can afford to hire a postpartum doula, you may find this kind of help invaluable.

Women who have had relatively short, easy labors sometimes try to resume their normal pace of life on the first few days following birth. Because they feel fit enough to go out to eat or cook a meal for the family, they often can't think of a good reason to slow their pace. But this expenditure of energy doesn't contribute to ease in nursing, as would sitting or lying still while holding the baby. I discourage too much activity during the first week or so after giving birth, because your body is going through enormous changes as you make the transition from pregnancy to lactation, and the process works much better when you are resting. Women who try to resume their normal activities during this first week often end up feeling exhausted and depressed. The boost in energy that you may feel after giving birth should be saved, not spent. If your postbirth bleeding slacks off and then gets heavier again, you are probably being too active.

Don't be surprised if your baby sleeps more in the daytime than at night. Most babies are born with the habit of being awake during the night; this likely has something to do with the fact that when you were asleep during the last weeks of pregnancy, your uterus was more relaxed and thus much roomier than when you were awake. You might as well give in to the idea that this habit isn't going to change right away and plan accordingly. You will need to learn to sleep when your baby sleeps—both day and night. It may be comforting to know that when you do get a chance to sleep, you probably won't have any problem doing so as soon as your head hits the pillow. The hormones associated with breastfeeding are the kind that help you fall asleep easily. If you still have trouble sleeping in the daytime, you can try using an eyeshade.

Emotionally, you may feel less than confident and, if your baby is not one of those who latch successfully on the first couple of attempts, you may even feel rejected by her. Will you feel that she doesn't like you? I hope not, but many women have reported such feelings. Few women today have had a chance to closely observe newborn babies nursing, and this lack keeps them from learning babies' cues and interpreting what they mean. Because of the invisibility of nursing in our society, many women believe that nursing a baby should be easy and almost automatic or that it is too much trouble to be worth trying. Both of these extreme views are imbalanced and inaccurate; in truth, many women say that the first two to three weeks were very challenging but that they were glad they persisted until they and their babies figured out how to do it right.

Ideally, the first priority of maternity-care policy-making is to make sure that such care truly and comprehensively meets the needs of women and their babies around the time of birth and the sensitive period thereafter. Good maternity care makes it possible for women to concentrate their full attention on their newborn babies, thereby increasing the chance for each mother to have a smooth transition into breastfeeding, reducing levels of postpartum depression, and minimizing chances of illnesses for both mother and baby during the first year following birth. In the Netherlands, the government health plan provides for a specially trained nurse/lactation expert to help each new baby's parents in their home for a full ten days following each birth (with a small co-payment). Hired for three, five, or eight hours according to individual families' needs, this maternity nurse serves the new parents breakfast in bed, feeds any older children their breakfast, walks the dog, helps the new mother with breastfeeding if necessary, cleans the house, and notifies the midwife if the mother or baby should need medical attention for any reason. The Dutch consider the care provided each family by the maternity nurse to be an investment in good health, which benefits the entire society because it so effectively reduces the number of illnesses mothers and babies experience during the first year of the baby's life and thus saves money budgeted for women and children's care.

Why should women in the United States put up with anything less?

6

PROBLEM-SOLVING DURING

THE FIRST WEEK

Engorgement

If both of your breasts feel hard, tight, and painful during the first week, and the skin of your breasts looks tight and shiny, but you don't have a fever (your temperature is less than 101 degrees F, or 38.4 degrees C), then your breasts are engorged. This is different from the normal swelling and fullness that is supposed to happen between days three and five after birth, when your breasts feel full but not painful and your nipples are still soft and pliable. With engorgement, this normal swelling becomes much more pronounced, to the point that the nipple and areola may be stretched so hard and tight that the baby has trouble grasping enough breast in his mouth to get a good latch.

Engorgement can look like mastitis—a bacterial breast infection—since both conditions involve swelling, but the two shouldn't be confused. While engorgement always involves both sides, mastitis usually happens on one side only. With engorgement, there is no infection, so there is no need for you to take antibiotics. The condition usually passes quickly, lasting only a day or two. You can lessen its severity by promptly taking the following steps, which will help reduce your symptoms and will allow your baby to get a good latch more easily.

- Soften your nipple and areola by manually expressing some milk.

- Once your breasts are soft enough for your baby to get a good latch, nurse as long and frequently as you can. The idea is to remove as much milk as possible, since doing so will reduce the amount of lymphatic fluid in your breasts, helping to reverse the engorgement.

- As your baby nurses, continuously press on the breast he is nursing from to help your milk flow to your nipple.

- Once your baby ends a feeding, express as much milk as possible, as this will lessen any pain or discomfort you feel. If it causes you to make more milk, this is good. You can store any that your baby doesn't take.

- Between feedings, apply cold compresses to your breasts for your comfort. Refrigerated cabbage leaves, cupped around each breast three or four times a day, can also be soothing.

- If you need pain relief for your letdown to happen, take some ibuprofen. It's a safe choice, because it reduces inflammation but won't have a negative effect on your baby.

- Keep up your own fluid intake. Drinking plenty of fluids won't aggravate engorgement.

It is usually possible to prevent engorgement by nursing your baby frequently during the first few days of life. Keep in mind that if you had an epidural there is a greater chance that you will have engorgement, because extra IV fluids are given with an epidural. It usually takes three or four days for your body to rid itself of this extra fluid load, some of which will be in your breasts, so you may find that you experience engorgement on the fourth or fifth day after your baby's birth.

Sore Nipples

Nipple soreness is not a condition that you should try to tolerate. You need to discover the cause of your nipple soreness so that you know what to do about it. Get help from a lactation consultant or peer counselor as soon as you notice it, unless you are able to ease the situation yourself right away.

The most common form of nipple soreness indicates that there is something wrong with the way your baby is latching or is positioned at your breast. This type of soreness is sharpest when your baby latches on and during a feeding. If you have soreness like this, it is likely that you have been allowing your baby to suck in a way that has traumatized your nipples. More incorrect sucking will only worsen the problem. Prolonged nipple soreness from a poor latch can lead to a cracked or bleeding nipple and even to mastitis (a bacterial breast infection). If your baby latches the right way, you should experience immediate relief. If this happens, continue nursing sessions until your baby decides to let go. Even if he wants to nurse for a long time, your sore nipples can heal if he is latched correctly.

Perhaps your baby's first few sucks are a bit painful but the pain subsides after your milk lets down. As long as your nipple doesn't look asymmetrical or misshapen just after a nursing session or have any pinkish or blistered areas, this kind of soreness shouldn't progress to something worse. Soreness of this kind is usually gone after a week has passed, given that the latch appears good and your baby is producing the required number of soaked diapers.

However, a nipple that looks misshapen or asymmetrical just after the baby lets go of it is a strong indication that your problem is a poor latch rather than passing soreness. The same goes for a nipple that has a water blister or an area that is pinkish or reddish.

Cracked or Bleeding Nipples

If your nipples are cracked or bleeding on one or both sides, and you have managed to achieve a good latch, it's a good idea to hand-express a little milk to soften your nipple before offering your breast. Use your less-sore side until your letdown happens and then switch to the more-sore side, making sure that the latch is good. When your baby has finished nursing, express a little milk or colostrum and let it dry on your nipple, as its antibacterial properties will help protect you from infection. I would also recommend that you use a thin layer of over-the-counter antibiotic ointment (Polysporin, for instance) for infection prevention when there is a break in your skin. Don't worry if your baby swallows any; the drug is quickly metabolized and is considered safe. You also needn't worry if your baby swallows blood from a damaged nipple. No harm will come to him.

The best way to avoid a scab from forming on a cracked or bleeding nipple is to keep it moist between feedings with Lansinoh brand lanolin. (You can apply this over the antibiotic ointment you're using.) La Leche League International recommends Lansinoh specifically for sore or cracked nipples, because, unlike some other lanolin brands, it contains no preservatives or additives. Use enough and apply it often enough to keep your nipple area from drying. Steer clear of products such as vitamin ointments, any petroleum-based products such as Vaseline, or anything with alcohol in it. You should also keep soaps and lotions away from your nipples. Any Lansinoh that is present on your nipple when a feeding begins will not harm your baby.

Here is another regimen for cracked nipples, offered by Canadian lactation expert and pediatrician Dr. Jack Newman. You'll need a doctor to prescribe it for you.

All-Purpose Nipple Ointment:

- Mupirocin 2 percent ointment (15 grams)
- Nystatin ointment, 100,000 units/milliliter (15 grams)
- Miconazole *powder* to a final concentration of 2 percent

The virtue of this ointment is that it contains antibiotic, antifungal, and steroidal ingredients, which makes it effective against most causes of sore nipples. You can mix up your own version of this ointment using hydrocortisone cream as the steroid, an antifungal such as Lotrimin, and an antibiotic ointment such as Neosporin. This ointment should be applied to your nipples right after feeding and shouldn't be wiped off. It will not hurt your baby to swallow any of it.

Lactation consultant Bonnie Reed uses a variation on this method that she finds very effective, particularly if she suspects that the cracked nipples are caused by a yeast infection. She advises affected mothers to use vinegar and water to rinse the milk sugar off the nipples after feeding sessions. (This is most easily done by mixing half vinegar and half water in a Ziploc bag with small squares of Viva paper towels.) After this, the all-purpose cream can be applied to the nipples.

If your cracked nipple is so painful that you dread your baby's next nursing session, you can take an over-the-counter pain medication such as acetaminophen an hour or so before you expect your baby to feed. You might also want to wrap some ice cubes in a washcloth and hold these to your nipple, as this will have a temporary numbing effect.

If your bra has become uncomfortable, leave it off while your nipples are healing, or choose a larger size. Apply Lansinoh or Dr. Jack Newman's ointment. If you get a larger bra, put a couple of breast shells or tea strainers (with the handles removed and the edges covered with soft adhesive tape) inside your bra to keep any pressure or friction away from your nipples. In general, your bra is too small if you find pressure marks on your breasts after wearing.

Nipple soreness can result from the improper use of a breast pump. See Chapter 8 for more information on breast pumps.

Some women also experience nipple soreness because of having extra-sensitive skin. A Dutch friend, Karin, tells her story:

Karin: *Nursing caused a lot of pain for me because of a skin condition I have. It is not psoriasis, although it is related to it. Mine is called "atopic eczema," which means it is a nondescript rash that can pop up anywhere. It comes with a very dry and sensitive skin. I tried all the usual cures and creams, to no avail. I called a lactation expert, as it hurt so much that after some weeks I was on the verge of giving up nursing, although I didn't really want to quit. She told me to try a breast pump for just a few days to give the skin time to heal, and that worked. Another thing that helped was that I always used just one breast at a time, so the other one could dry and rest. I sat around bare-breasted a lot of the time. When I had to get dressed, I used tea strainers. This keeps the*

fabric away from the skin and allows air in. The skin just needs more time to recover, and if you can find a way to give it a chance to do that, it'll get firmer and your condition will improve. At any rate, I continued breastfeeding for a year and a half after that bout of soreness with no problem.

Painless Bleeding from the Breast

Sometimes during late pregnancy or the first week following birth, you may experience painless bleeding from your nipples. This condition usually clears up within a few days and is not harmful to you or your baby. It is sometimes called "rusty-pipe syndrome," a term that is probably meant to ease the alarm and worry that rust-colored milk often causes. If bleeding from the nipples continues for more than two weeks, see a doctor to determine the cause.

Yeast or Thrush Infection

An entire category of nipple soreness is caused by a fungal overgrowth called thrush—the same organism that you have in a vaginal yeast infection (*Candida albicans*). Thrush infections can occur at any time during the nursing period.

Signs and symptoms that you have thrush include:

- Burning pain or itchiness of the nipples.

- Tiny white spots on the nipples.

- Sudden-onset pain despite an obvious good latch and positioning.

- Shooting pain during or after feedings, moving from chest to nipples.

- Pain despite no visible signs of nipple soreness, such as blistering, pinkness, or a distorted shape of the nipple.

- Vaginal yeast infection.

Signs of thrush in your baby include:

- White patches inside his mouth on his cheeks, gums, tongue, or the back of his throat. These patches will look sore underneath if you rub the white patch off. (If the white is on his tongue only, it's probably not thrush.)
- Red, raised rash on his bottom.
- Clicking sounds while nursing, breast refusal, or repeated pulling away from the breast after having latched. This is a strong sign of yeast infection even if there are no white patches.

Thrush should be treated quickly in both you and your baby, as this is the only way to keep you from reinfecting each other. Thrush is quite painful for the mother, but it's not always painful for the baby (although it can be), so it can be difficult to tell if he's infected. If you have the symptoms, it is necessary to treat your baby as well, even if he exhibits no symptoms at all.

Thrush infections often occur after oral or IV antibiotics are taken, because antibiotics kill not only the harmful bacteria but also those that are needed to maintain the healthy balance of flora in the body. They are more common in women with diabetes or a history of vaginal yeast infections and in those who use corticosteroids for asthma, whose diets include a lot of dairy products, fruits, and sweeteners (both natural and artificial), and those who use nursing pads or plastic-lined bras.

Treating Thrush

Let's start with a home remedy. Add one teaspoon of bicarbonate of soda (baking soda) to one cup of water that has been boiled for twenty minutes. It's best to keep this mixture in a tightly sealed jar so you can use it whenever and wherever necessary for several days. The mixture can be applied to your nipples and your baby's mouth (and hands) using a gauze pad, a cotton applicator, or a clean cloth soaked with the solution.

Treatment with gentian violet is also an effective and inexpensive—

although messy—way to treat a yeast infection. It works quickly, and you can use it on your baby, yourself, and your partner (who, without treatment, may keep you infected through sexual contact). You can buy gentian violet over the counter at a pharmacy. You will want a one percent dilution. Most of the gentian violet that is available is two percent, so you can dilute it by half with sterile water. Apply the purple solution with a cotton-tipped applicator on all of the surfaces where the yeast may have taken up residence. (Be sure to put away any clothes, sheets, or diapers that you don't want purpled, as this is very staining.) If your nipples aren't purple after a feeding, apply more until they are. Another good way to get the gentian violet into your baby's mouth is to apply it generously to your breast and then nurse your baby. If you see purple milk, don't worry—it's harmless. The good thing about gentian violet is that it will usually do away with a yeast infection within a couple of days. Repeat the treatment once a day for four days. If the pain continues beyond this time, the problem may be something other than thrush, and it would be wise for you to get good help from a pediatrician who is knowledgeable about breastfeeding.

If you wish to avoid the purple treatment, and the candida infection hasn't become well entrenched, you might try homeopathic calendula ointment, which you can obtain at any health-food store that carries homeopathic remedies.

Some women have found other ways to quiet down an overgrowth of yeast. These include:

- Taking acidophilus bifidus (400 million to one billion viable units per day) for at least two weeks after symptoms disappear.

- Taking grapefruit-seed extract (250 mg three times per day, or five to fifteen drops in five ounces of water two to five times daily).

- Taking garlic tablets (three triple-strength tablets, three times per day for two weeks or more), zinc (45 mg daily), and B vitamins (100 mg of each from any source besides nutritional yeast).

- Eating a cup of live cultured yogurt (unsweetened is best) per day.

Another, more expensive option is a prescription product called Nystatin suspension. Nystatin should be used after every feeding for at least two weeks. It's useful to know that at least one study found it less effective at treating thrush than several other options.

When thrush keeps coming back, and nursing pain continues after other treatments, you might want to try a prescription cream called Diflucan (fluconazole).

Whatever form of treatment you choose, continue breastfeeding your baby; there is no reason to stop. You should rinse your nipples often as you treat for thrush, but avoid soaping them (do, however, frequently wash your hands with soap and water). Wear a clean bra each day and also change the hand towels you use daily. Remember that damp breast pads and wet sheets near your breasts can help to nurture the yeast cells whose growth you don't want to encourage. Wash your baby's hands if he sucks his thumbs or fingers. Any toys that have been in your baby's mouth should be washed in hot, soapy water and rinsed well. Remember that whatever treatment you choose, your partner will need to receive the treatment as well.

Plugged Milk Duct

If you develop a lump or a tender spot in your breast without a fever or flulike symptoms, it is likely to be a plugged milk duct, which means that milk is no longer moving freely through that part of your breast. This causes inflammation and soreness, which usually affects only one breast at a time. Plugged milk ducts are often caused by bras that are too tight, so if this might be the case with you, it would be wise to go bra-less, at least for several days. Some nursing mothers who sleep on their bellies find that this position can cause a plugged duct. In general, you should watch out for any pressure that you might be putting on your breast that could restrict the milk flow, whether it is from constrictive clothing, wearing or wrapping a baby too tightly at the breast, carrying a bag with straps that put pressure on a portion of your breast, your older baby biting you, or using too small a flange or the wrong pressure setting on your breast pump. Dehydration can also contribute to a plugged duct, so make sure that you cut down your caffeine intake and drink enough water.

When you have a plugged duct, it is essential for you to keep feeding your baby from the affected breast. The flow of milk through the congested part of your breast—the stronger the flow, the better—will help to prevent the more serious and painful problem of mastitis. (If you have recurrent plugged ducts, you are more likely to experience an episode of mastitis.)

Vary nursing positions, as long as your baby is able to latch well from each position used, and pay attention to see if a position that is different from the one you usually use helps to soften the sore area. I've seen a blocked milk duct get fixed when the mother knelt over her baby, who was lying on his back with his legs extended toward his mother's head. Though you shouldn't do anything that is painful or uncomfortable, be as creative as you want in working out alternative positions. The closer his lower jaw is to the plugged duct, the greater the chance that his sucking will remove the blockage.

Put a warm compress on the sore area or soak in a warm bath for ten minutes or so three times a day, then nurse your baby while your breast is still warm. Try massaging the sore area gently, using a circular motion at first, moving from above the sore area toward your nipple. Combine these movements with the compression that is always good to use when you want maximum milk flow to get to your baby.

A blocked milk duct is not a bacterial breast infection and therefore needs no treatment with antibiotics. If you need pain medication, ibuprofen is a good choice, as it can relieve inflammation as well as pain. For greatest effect, take it an hour before you anticipate a feeding.

Some women get a milk blister (bleb) along with a blocked duct. This is a white blister on the end of the nipple that contains some thickened milk. If it's quite painful, you can open it yourself (after a feeding) by using a sewing needle that you've sterilized in a flame. Squeeze out any fluid from behind the blister to keep it from re-forming, and prevent an infection by applying a topical antibiotic ointment such as Polysporin on that spot for a week after feedings.

Here's how one mother, June, solved the blocked-duct problem she experienced with her seventeen-month-old son:

June: *My son, Malik, still nurses at night. The night before last, I woke up at around five A.M. and realized he was asleep but still attached to my breast. It felt uncomfortable, and I picked him up and moved him up to pillow level, without taking him off properly. He usually pops right off when he's asleep, but this time his mouth didn't open, and as I pulled him off, his bottom teeth made a small cut on my nipple. OUCH! I was*

in pain and stayed in bed for a few hours trying to fall back asleep, without any luck.

That little injury affected me all through the next day, with extreme soreness on the nipple, especially when he was nursing. I didn't want to slow down feeding on that side, so I really had to just deal with the pain, hoping to prevent engorgement. The following morning I woke up with a hard lump at the top of my breast. I noticed it was becoming painful, and I lay in bed dreading the worst: that it would worsen into mastitis. I knew I had to get out of bed and take care of it right away. I was pretty sure that this was a blocked duct, so I spent the morning trying everything I could think of to help move it through. I tried running hot water on the area, I took some ibuprofen to help with inflammation, I tried to hand-express the milk out, and when Malik nursed, I tried to angle him so that his chin was directly on the clogged duct. Nothing seemed to help, and the lump seemed to get bigger and more painful.

After almost an hour soaking in a hot bath and using the shower spray with hot water directly on the sore area, I noticed something when I was hand-expressing. There was a small white dot that appeared only when I was squeezing the milk out. Milk was coming from the other nipple pores but not from this one small white dot. It suddenly occurred to me that this was where the milk was being redirected, since the milk could not exit where the small cut was healing over.

I asked my husband for a needle, and he brought me a small sterile lancet. I carefully pricked the little white dot, and milk came out in a perfect stream. Holding my breast like a sandwich and rolling my fingers and thumbs a few inches down toward the nipple, I hand-expressed for three to five minutes and watched streams of milk come out almost exclusively from this nipple pore. The other milk ducts were empty from the nursing and hand-expressing that had already taken place. After these few minutes, the hard lump was gone, and I felt an extreme sense of relief.

Mastitis

Mastitis is caused by bacteria—usually *Staphylococcus aureus*—that take up residence in your breast. It's easier to develop an infection if you have a sore or cracked nipple, if your immune system is weakened, if engorgement leads to such fullness in your breasts that your letdown reflex isn't happening, if a plugged duct isn't resolved, if you are going through a time of high stress and extreme fatigue, or even if your genetic inheritance gave you especially thin skin.

Symptoms of mastitis include a sore spot or lump in your breast that is hot to touch, chills and fever (more than 101 degrees F, or 38.4 degrees C), and/or flulike symptoms. Keep in mind, though, that these symptoms could also indicate that you have the flu and nothing more than a painful blocked duct. You will have a better idea that your problem is mastitis if your breast is also red and swollen, with or without red streaks (note: These symptoms do not occur in all women with mastitis).

An increased susceptibility toward mastitis runs in some families. If you have family members who have had a history of recurrent bouts of mastitis, though, you shouldn't be discouraged from breastfeeding. With experience, you will learn how your body functions and develop a list of strategies that will help you quickly recover from mastitis or even ward it off preemptively. Incidentally, if susceptibility to mastitis runs in your family, you might want to invest in a good electric breast pump to fight engorgement.

If you think that you have mastitis, you should respond immediately to its early symptoms—there are several steps you can take over the next twenty-four hours to improve your condition and to shorten your illness. I've listed below the steps that I've found to be most effective.

- Follow all the steps for curing a plugged milk duct (see pages 131–132).

- Make sure that all your family members understand your needs and know how to help you; you'll need help with housework and meals and will need someone to care for any older children that you may have. This will allow you to get all the rest you need.

- Apply heat to the sorest part of your breast, and massage the affected area gently.

- Take twenty to forty drops of echinacea (purple coneflower) tincture six times during the first day of symptoms. You can add it to water if you like. If this treatment seems to be working, follow these instructions: On days two through five, drink two glasses of

water, each containing a half drop of echinacea tincture for every pound of your body weight. On days six through ten, drink one glass of this tincture–water mixture each day. Though echinacea tincture is easier for most people to obtain than echinacea root, herbalist Susun Weed prefers to treat mastitis with echinacea infusions, prepared in the following manner: Steep one ounce of the root per pint of boiling water for at least eight hours. Drink two cups daily until the fever comes down. Then make a lighter infusion, with one ounce of the root per quart of boiling water, and drink one to two cups daily for an additional week.

- Contact your lactation consultant, physician, or midwife. You will likely be prescribed an antibiotic. It's good to have this on hand in case the echinacea remedy doesn't substantially improve your symptoms during the next twenty-four hours. You should try the echinacea tincture first, though, because it is an herbal treatment. Unlike a prescription antibiotic, it won't create the conditions for a thrush infection.

- Apply a poultice of parsley or comfrey directly to your breast. Here's how: Wrap a handful of fresh or dried parsley in a clean cotton cloth, tie it with a string or rubber band, and steep it in simmering water for ten to fifteen minutes. Let the parcel cool to the point where you can tolerate it directly on your breast.

- Keep a bottle of hand sanitizer near you and wash your hands before each nursing session. Clean any phones, remote devices, or other items that you handle as well, so you minimize chances of reinfecting yourself.

While you are treating mastitis, you should continue breastfeeding frequently from the affected breast, whether you are taking an antibiotic or an herbal medicine. It may take as long as twenty-four to forty-eight hours before some of your symptoms subside. Your milk will not hurt your baby—even if there is a little blood in it—and the suction will help your condition.

Women can sometimes fight off a threatened bout of mastitis by heeding the early warning signs during the twenty-four hours after the first appearance of symptoms. Echinacea can be taken preventively: ten

to fifteen drops of tincture in a glass of water twice a day for a minimum of five days.

Poor Tongue Habits

Some babies have trouble sucking effectively because they have developed tongue habits that interfere with a good latch—for example, a baby may suck his tongue, push the nipple out of his mouth with his tongue, hold his tongue in the back of his mouth, or curl its tip upward. Any one of these habits can keep him from drawing the breast far enough back into his mouth to be able to get milk. One sign that he is using his tongue incorrectly is a vertical red strip on your nipple and a feeling that he's chewing instead of sucking.

If any poor tongue habit has become ingrained, you may need the help of a lactation consultant to solve the problem, but when a baby is less than a week old, it's often possible to help him learn how to use his tongue correctly.

The baby who keeps his tongue in the back of his mouth can sometimes be coaxed to drop his tongue and bring it forward if you brush your breast lightly across his lips. Bring him to the breast as soon as you see the lowered, extended tongue and open mouth. Patience and precision timing are needed to teach your baby a new habit.

If your baby clenches his lips tightly during a feeding session, it's best not to keep pushing him. You don't want to give him a negative experience when you are trying to teach something important. Rocking your baby gently can help to relax his mouth and tongue, as well as his body. Once he is well relaxed, it's good to try nursing again. Begin by manually expressing a little colostrum and getting some on his lips or tongue. Once he gapes well, cuddle him to you so he can reach your breast.

If your baby retracts his tongue and uses it to push against your nipple, you should put gentle pressure on the middle part of his tongue with your clean finger (cut your fingernail first, please) until his tongue begins to cup your finger. Dripping some of your milk into his mouth may also help him bring his tongue down and forward into the proper position. Rock your baby gently to relax him and then brush his lips with your breast, pulling him toward or away from your breast according to whether he is opening his mouth wide and dropping his tongue low (pull

toward) or giving you a more pursed mouth with his tongue held high or sticking out slightly (pull away). You need to observe him closely as you do this and respond to his changes immediately. Be patient with him as he learns.

The Tongue-Tied Baby

An easily solved problem that is frequently missed during the first days of a newborn's life is when the frenulum is too tight to permit effective suckling—in popular language, this condition is called "tongue-tie." The frenulum is the thin membrane under the tongue that attaches the tongue to the bottom of the mouth and keeps us from swallowing our tongues. When it's too tight, it doesn't permit the baby enough free movement of the tongue to allow his lips to curl around the areola, making a good seal. A tongue-tied baby can't extend his tongue past his lower lip. Many babies with this condition quickly hurt their mothers' nipples enough to lead to several problems with breastfeeding, which may include injured nipples and infection of the breast for you and too little milk, trouble swallowing, and a slow weight gain for your baby. Tongue-tie runs in families and occurs in about one to five percent of all babies. It's important to know that tight frenula rarely fix themselves, so this is a problem you should address promptly if you notice that it is preventing your baby from nursing properly.

Tongue-tie occurs in varying degrees of severity. In severe cases, the tongue is heart-shaped instead of coming to a point at the end. In more moderate cases, the frenulum may look less tight toward the end of the tongue but still be tight enough farther back to keep the tongue from cupping the breast well when the baby attempts to latch—when this happens, your baby will get little milk for his efforts. In more-minor cases of tongue-tie, babies are sometimes able to grasp and draw their mothers' nipples back into their mouths and thus have no problem suckling.

Babies who don't get the reward of milk soon become frustrated with or tired of nursing. Some will begin to clamp their gums together onto their mothers' sensitive nipples, causing pain and injury (this will also decrease the stimulation of milk flow); others will express their frustration by arching away from the breast. Though the tongue-tied baby

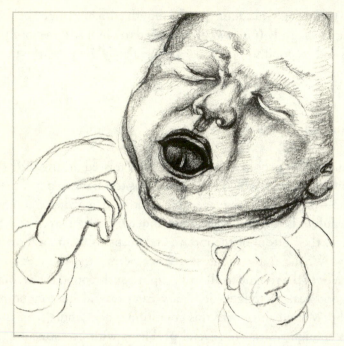

The tongue-tied baby

may appear to have a good latch, he will probably not be getting enough milk from you to prosper. If your baby seems well latched but is fussy and unsettled during feedings, check him for tongue-tie. A baby who gets enough milk at the breast will relax his entire body once the milk begins to flow well and he is busily feeding. A baby who is working hard at the breast while getting little reward will remain tense.

The remedy for tongue-tie is to snip the frenulum. This used to be a common procedure that a family physician, midwife, or pediatrician completed in a few seconds. I remember my mentor, Dr. John O. Williams, Jr., explaining to my midwife partner and me how this was the easiest thing a doctor or midwife could do, with the biggest reward, in the shortest amount of time. The cut itself is close to painless (less so than ear piercing) and ordinarily involves no more than a drop or two of blood (although the baby might cry from being held still). The benefits are instant; the baby can take the breast after the cut is made. While most babies will be able to latch on immediately, some others may have to be encouraged to stick their tongues out before they can suckle effectively.

Oddly, the trouble that many women with tongue-tied babies encounter is that their pediatricians refuse to snip the frenulum, because they see no point in performing this simple procedure and are ignorant of the possible negative impact tongue-tie can have on breastfeeding. Lactation consultants often disagree with pediatricians in these cases, but, even though they know more about nursing, they may be outranked by the pediatricians.

When a short frenulum is discovered on the first day or two, it's not necessary to do anything—as long as your nipples aren't sore and your baby seems to be getting enough milk. Your baby may be one of the lucky few whose tight frenulum stretches enough as he moves it to allow for successful breastfeeding. But if your nipples are sore during the first week after birth (even though your baby's latch looks good) and your baby's frenulum makes it hard for his tongue to reach his lips, you should seek the opinion of your lactation consultant. If your lactation consultant and your pediatrician disagree, I recommend that you continue to work with your lactation consultant to find a doctor or dentist to make the snip.

Candace's story shows what a miraculous difference snipping the frenulum can have on tongue-tied babies.

Candace: *My twin girls were born strong and healthy, after an easy labor. I felt high with the magnificence of the whole experience and thought all my worries were over.*

Anna nursed quite vigorously. I found the sensation horribly unpleasant, but I let her stay on for about an hour. When she came off the breast, my nipple was deformed. Over the next thirty-six hours I repeatedly asked for instructions to get a comfortable latch, but my doula, Carla, and the nurses thought the latch looked correct. I delivered on a weekend, so there was no lactation consultant on duty.

My first night home went well; the babies weren't particularly hungry. I nursed throughout the following day but felt things weren't quite right. My babies never relaxed. That evening all hell broke loose as the babies screamed in desperation while I tried to figure out how to get them latched on. By the end of this eight-hour ordeal, they had developed an aversion to my breasts and were limp and silent with exhaustion. I felt unfathomable despair.

I had an appointment with their pediatrician that afternoon and hoped he would be able to instruct me. I tried many more times to nurse the babies, but they had given up on feeding. Before we left for their checkup, I expressed about an ounce of colostrum, which I divided and poured into each of their mouths.

While waiting to see our pediatrician, I felt my milk come in. When the nurse weighed the babies, she found that they had lost seventeen percent of their birth weight. The pediatrician came in and informed us that the babies were malnourished and jaundiced. He told me that while he was for breastfeeding, he was not for breastfeeding to the detriment of any infant. (I'd never heard of deleterious effects of breastfeeding before!) He said I didn't have enough milk for twins and gave me some formula. He told me that he would give me forty-eight hours to turn their health around, or he would admit them to the hospital.

Driving home I felt horrible, but I was informed enough to know that the doctor was wrong about my milk supply. I knew that the volume of milk I could produce was as yet untested, since flow hadn't been established. At home the babies drank formula, courtesy of their grandparents, while I sat down and figured out how to use the electric pump we had bought in preparation of my eventual return to work. I pumped continuously for the next forty-eight hours, stopping only to feed the babies what I extracted.

At first, the amount I made closely matched the amount the babies were able to eat. It started out at about one ounce per side, then increased to one and a half, then two and so on, and the babies kept up until about three and a half ounces. By day two my supply far outstripped the size of the babies' stomachs, and by day three I could extract fourteen ounces every two hours. I fed them two to three ounces every two to three hours and stored the surplus in the freezer. When we returned to the pediatrician, the babies had gained about six ounces each.

I asked him how I could get the babies to suckle and he told me to call the hospital lactation nurse. We met, and after three hours it became quite clear that my problems weren't as simple as latch and position. She did teach me, however, not to hold the back of the baby's head to the breast—which causes her to resist in fear of being smothered—but to support the neck where it meets with the shoulder so that when a baby wants, she is free to move her head as she pleases. At my two-week postnatal checkup, I described my breastfeeding difficulties to the midwife, and she called an independent lactation consultant, Hannah, for me.

Hannah came over to my house that week, and after another three hours had both babies latched on and nursing. However, even though we had the best latch possible, it was still quite painful. Hannah convinced me to call a chiropractic office that specialized in cranial–sacral therapy for newborns. She pointed out that Anna's head was stuck in a flexed position and that she was scowling as if in pain, even during sleep. Anna's head was compressed at the temples, causing the cranium to bulge. She explained how these situations interfered with the full range of jaw movement that a baby needs to breastfeed well.

When my twins were six weeks old, Hannah called me and asked if I would bring the girls to an in-service at the chiropractic office, since they were the youngest patients in the practice and she wanted to have babies of all ages. The girls would receive a free treatment and be evaluated by the teaching physician, Dr. Coryllos. Hannah explained that Dr. Coryllos had just completed a five-year study on the effects of tongue-tie. Hannah said that it was unlikely that my girls had tongue-tie but that the physicians attending the in-service would get to practice diagnosing the disorder on other babies who would be present.

I went and spent the first half of the day listening to a fascinating lecture on tongue-tie and its effects on babies' facial development, nursing ability, digestion, speech pathology, and how it feels to the breastfeeding mother. Many mothers said it was like being licked by a cat's tongue. I perked up because that described my experience perfectly.

Also, because it is such hard work for a baby to compensate and nurse with tongue-tie, she takes longer to feed, becomes exhausted, and then must nurse again soon after, sometimes within fifteen minutes. When Dr. Coryllos examined my infants, she found that they both had posterior tongue-ties, the most difficult kind to diagnose, since it's deep in the flesh of the tongue just behind the salivary glands. All the physicians crowded around my babies' mouths with interest.

The doctor then demonstrated the procedure on another infant. The infant was swaddled and held firmly on his back by four pairs of hands while the physician used a dental tool to expose the tight frenulum. Orajel was applied and the frenulum clipped with a small blunt-tipped scissors. A two-inch square of cotton gauze was applied to the cut for no less than two minutes to stanch any bleeding. [Posterior tongue-ties tend to bleed more than the common kind of tongue-tie.] The baby was then put to his mother's breast.

Dr. Coryllos invited my babies to be her demonstration patients at an in-service the following day. Both had the procedure. Not only was I able to exclusively breastfeed, but their growth rocketed, since they were now getting my hindmilk. A breast pump doesn't extract fatty hindmilk nearly as efficiently as a baby does.

Since this happened, I ask every little kid I talk with to stick their tongue out for me. When I see a tongue-tie, which is quite often, I ask the mother if she nursed her baby. A couple of them were able to, but most say that they didn't enjoy breastfeeding, it was painful, or they didn't think they had enough milk because the baby was never full. I don't judge women who say they couldn't breastfeed anymore, because I know that it can break your heart. Looking back, I spent the majority of my time and energy preparing for labor and making sure I was able to deliver twins safely and naturally. The birthing was a nonissue, but I did labor long and hard to breastfeed. It, too, was worth it.

The Baby Who Needs More Fluid

In general, young babies get all of their fluid requirements from breast-feeding. It is possible, though, for a baby to become dehydrated enough to upset his electrolyte balance. In this case, it can be a good idea to give a very young baby supplemental liquid.

Here is an example of what I mean: I was once asked to examine a young baby (five or six days old) who was born to an Old Order Amish woman during an extreme Tennessee heat wave. The baby's mother was worried because, instead of waking during the day to feed, as all her other babies had, her new son slept all day long, waking to feed only two or three times at night. The family lived in a small cottage with a metal roof in a yard with no shade, and the Old Order Amish still dress their babies as if they were born in northern Europe, in long-sleeved dresses and bonnets, regardless of season.

When I arrived, I could see right away what the problem was. His clothes were damp with sweat from the intense heat in the house, and he was dehydrated and lethargic. Because there was no electricity in the house, there was no way to set up a fan. To solve the problem, I recommended that the baby be dressed in clothing light enough that he didn't sweat (in his case, a diaper only), and we gave him two ounces (60 g) of an electrolyte as a temporary measure. This combination proved enough to return the baby to a more normal pattern of waking every two to three hours to suckle, night and day.

The Baby Who Arches Away from the Breast

Some babies have such great muscle tension that they have trouble staying on the breast once latched. Instead of curling forward as babies usually do in cradle hold, they arch their head and upper body away from the breast. Babies like this are more likely to hold their legs extended, rather than to flex them at the knees and hips. They suck a few times and then let go before they can fall into a regular pattern of sucking and swallowing. It may help to rock the tense baby into a calmer state of mind before introducing him to the breast again. Some tense babies eat more effectively when they are sleepy than when they are alert and wide awake. It often helps to hold a tense baby belly-down on your lap and gently massage his back to help him calm down before bringing him to the breast. This baby may relax and nurse better while lying on top of you. Swaddling may prove helpful in getting him to relax before nursing.

7

SLEEPING ARRANGEMENTS

Where is your new baby going to sleep? A generation ago, you probably would have found a bassinet and a crib and thought little more about it. Now you may be trying to decide whether you should keep your baby in bed with you at night (called bed-sharing, co-sleeping, or the family bed) or put her to sleep in a bassinet or crib. Which way is better? There's no easy answer to this question—different solutions work better for different families.

Emotions sometimes run high surrounding the choices parents make about the sleeping arrangements for their young babies, just as they do about the choice between nursing and the feeding of substitute formulas. Proponents of one sleeping style sometimes become so judgmental about the other choice that they act as if those who make different decisions couldn't possibly be good parents. In reality, some parents begin sleeping with their babies, only to later find out that co-sleeping doesn't suit either them or the baby (and vice versa).

Babies are unique little beings, each with her own personality and needs. There may be differences within the same family; some families find out that the sleeping arrangement that worked for one of their babies does not suit a younger sibling or that an arrangement that worked well for a young baby needs to be changed as the baby grows older. For this reason, I recommend that you do your best to keep an open mind as you think about which style most appeals to you (and your spouse or partner) and then be flexible enough to change if your first choice doesn't work out.

Proponents of co-sleeping maintain that it makes breastfeeding easier (a claim that is undisputed, by the way) during the early weeks, when new parents are most exhausted. They also believe that it creates a more trusting relationship between parents and babies because it keeps babies from suffering from feelings of abandonment during the night. Other benefits include:

- Better sleep for mother and baby.

- A reduced risk of sudden infant death syndrome, when the principles of safe co-sleeping are followed.

- Women who return to jobs outside their homes and are separated from their babies for much of the day often feel that sleeping together helps them regain a strong sense of connection with the baby (and also helps them keep up their milk supply).

On the other hand, those who promote putting babies to sleep in bassinets or cribs also say that their favored sleeping arrangement reduces the risk of sudden infant death syndrome, helps mothers and babies sleep better, and teaches babies good sleeping habits.

We'll look more closely at the safety information for both of these arrangements, but first I want to point out that it's generally safer for your baby to sleep lying on her back or side than to be tummy-down, whether in the family bed or in a crib or bassinet. There is agreement that putting young babies to sleep on their backs cuts the risk of suffocation or strangulation. Statistics from several countries that have promoted babies sleeping on their backs show significantly lowered rates of sudden infant death syndrome since these programs began in the late 1980s. Of course, there are some babies who object to sleeping on their backs, who will put up quite a fuss until they are placed on their tummies to sleep. If you have one of these, you'll have to use your best judgment as to what works better for your particular situation.

Some parents worry that a baby who vomits while lying on her back might choke in this position. Babies with gastric reflux disease shouldn't be placed on their backs to sleep, precisely because they do vomit so frequently.

Safety Information for Co-Sleepers

If you have read much about co-sleeping, you or your relatives may have encountered some of the negative publicity that has been given to this sleeping arrangement. The American Academy of Pediatrics (AAP)—specifically the AAP's Task Force on Sudden Infant Death Syndrome—made a policy statement in 2005 saying that co-sleeping is hazardous to babies. The Canadian Paediatric Society also recommends that babies sleep in cribs placed in the parents' room for at least the first six months of life. The AAP task force based its recommendation upon a survey of all the sudden infant death syndrome cases recorded in New Jersey between 1996 and 2000, in which the researchers collected information on bed-sharing status, lifestyle factors, sleeping position, and type of bed environment. Tellingly, most of the bed-sharing sudden infant deaths for which they found data involved unsafe sleeping positions (babies sleeping on tummies rather than on their backs), mothers who were smokers or drug users, and low-income mothers in homeless shelters that lacked safe sleeping environments for babies. In the latter cases, some of the mothers were sleeping on a couch with the baby and one or more older children.

It's also worth noting that not all pediatricians heed the recommendations made by the AAP with regard to raising their own children. Dr. William Sears, for instance, has written extensively about how his wife and some of their eight children taught him how much value co-sleeping can have for many families. There is obviously a lot of difference between responsible co-sleeping and the kind of unplanned co-sleeping that is likely to have influenced the policy statements mentioned above.

The safety of co-sleeping with a very young or small baby is dependent upon several factors. It's not for:

- Parents who are heavy sleepers.

- Parents who are smokers.

- Parents who drink alcohol.

- Parents who are very obese.

- Parents who sleep with older children or pets.

- Parents who are under the influence of any drug or medication that interferes with their awareness and ability to be awakened.

- Babysitters.

Each of these factors raises the risk of accidental suffocation and asphyxiation of a baby, particularly during the first six months of life. For this reason, it's a good idea to have a crib that you can use for those nights when you or your partner have had something alcoholic to drink or are sleeping more soundly than usual for whatever reason.

Co-sleeping is nothing new; it has almost certainly been the predominant mode in human sleeping patterns over time. What has changed a lot over time is the way that adults in urbanized cultures sleep. Wherever it is practiced, safe co-sleeping requires the right kind of bed environment.

Avoid the following:

- Sleeping on a couch with your baby.

- Sleeping on a bed with loose sheets, duvets, covers, or scattered pillows.

- Sleeping on a waterbed or soft mattress.

- Sleeping on a mattress with a crack between it and the wall in which a baby can become wedged.

- Sleeping under an electric blanket.

- Having a headboard or footboard on your bed in which the baby's head could get caught.

- Placing your bed near a window-shade cord or curtain in which a baby could become entangled.

It's also a good idea to avoid a mattress set on a frame if there is any possibility that the baby could become caught between the mattress and the frame. For this reason, some parents choose to put their mattress directly on the floor, in the middle of the bedroom. This latter option has advantages when your baby becomes older and begins to roll over, scoot, and crawl, because the fall to the floor will be only a few inches, compared to the two- to three-foot fall from the average bed you are likely to find in a furniture store.

Keep in mind that your baby shouldn't be put to sleep alone on your bed. If she needs to go to sleep before you are ready to sleep with her, put her first in a crib and then move her when you are ready to go to bed.

Don't overdress your baby if you plan to co-sleep. It's quite easy for a baby to overheat while sleeping with an adult, since adults give off a lot of body heat. If you are interested in co-sleeping with your baby but are worried that you might sleep too soundly, there are several products now available that are designed to protect a small baby from suffocation. Two examples are a crib that can be fastened next to your mattress and a portable crib that can be placed in your bed. You can improvise one of these arrangements yourself by attaching your baby's crib to your bed with bungee cords.

Another option is to buy an enclosed hammock that can be hung just above your side of the bed. This allows for easy nursing, because you can untie the knot, lower the hammock to your level for feeding and soothing, and then raise the hammock back up, tying the knot at whatever height you like best. This arrangement also allows you to rock your baby if she isn't quite settled enough to sleep. I remember seeing many Chinese babies in Malaysia who were put to sleep in small hammocks like this. Once you have the hammock, you'll need a frame above your bed, a pulley, a rope, and a peg. This is usually an inexpensive arrangement to set up.

When Co-Sleeping Isn't So Easy

There is no doubt that co-sleeping turns out to be a completely satisfactory arrangement for many, many families and does live up to the claims made by its most fervent proponents. However, it doesn't seem to work for everyone. For some families, the reality of co-sleeping doesn't measure up to the ideal. Some babies and parents just sleep better when they have some distance between them, especially as the baby grows older. Problems sometimes arise because of a lack of true or continuing agreement between the baby's parents about co-sleeping. If your partner begins to complain about co-sleeping, it's important that you talk together so you can understand what is bothering him about the arrangement. It may be that you and the baby are doing fine, but Dad is beginning to wonder if he'll ever get any attention, loving, or sleep again. Maybe you and your partner can't get in the mood with the baby right there in your bed; perhaps you're afraid that you might wake your sleeping little one. Of course, finding places other than the bedroom for lovemaking can solve this problem, though spontaneity often has to give way to planning and scheduling some time together (especially when you have only fifteen minutes here and there). Whatever the problem is, solving it so that everyone's feelings are taken into account is a must.

Night Crawlers, Thrashers, and Kickers

As babies grow older, co-sleeping parents are sometimes presented with challenges they hadn't anticipated. The same baby who slept for longer stretches during the first weeks of life when close to her mother's body may begin to exhibit different behavior after a few short months. She may become an active night crawler who wakes everyone up to play for an hour or two during your prime sleeping hours. When this happens four or five times a night and things need to get done the next day, even the most patient mother may start reviewing her choices. It's one thing to have sleepless nights when your baby is less than four months or so old, when her stomach capacity is relatively small and she needs to eat more frequently than older children do. It's another situation when an attention habit, not hunger, is what drives her to wake up. The eight- or nine-month-old baby who nurses during the night and then falls back to sleep is not a problem. It's the one who keeps parents awake for hours on end during the night by fighting sleep when satiated.

Some babies escalate the amount of cuddling attention they want during the night. Nursing two or three times no longer suffices; now the baby calms down and goes to sleep only when held on Mom's chest after a nighttime feeding. If Mom obliges by becoming the human pillow for a rather heavy child, the ante goes up, and sometimes she won't settle for less than sleeping across Mom's throat. That is what I mean by an attention habit. Another variation on this theme is the baby who lets you know that it's time to wake up by sitting on your head. Even if these antics seem cute at first, how cute will they be as your baby gets heavier and heavier? How will you respond? Remember, if you give your baby affection (the breast) when she can't be hungry and she's doing something you'd rather she didn't do, you will be reinforcing this behavior, which means that you'll be likely to get more of it. The most important thing is that you are responsive to your baby when she needs you—not that she must be in constant contact with your body throughout the night in order to feel secure enough to sleep.

Some parents who think that their frisky baby will miss sleeping in their bed find out that she sleeps quite well once she is transferred to a crib. Babies who initially put up a fuss about sleeping anywhere besides the family bed can come to prefer sleeping in a crib and may even sleep more soundly alone.

If the thought of putting your scooting, thrashing baby into a crib doesn't work for you, you might try swaddling her first. Rambunctious babies between the ages of about four to seven months will often settle down and sleep much better if swaddled.

I believe that gradual changes generally work better than sudden ones. Let's say that your thriving older baby is used to falling asleep at your breast and you want to move her to her own space for sleeping. You might begin by first teaching her how to fall asleep without nursing. One way is to give just a short feed at bedtime, lie down with her, and then turn out the light while she's still awake. Tell her it's time to go to sleep and then refrain from interacting with her. If she's used to falling asleep around this time, she'll probably do so even without your breast in her mouth. Don't worry if she crawls around a little before this happens. Just calm yourself and keep from stirring her up in any way.

The next step in this sequence is to repeat these actions, and, once she's asleep in your bed, move her into her new bed (which you should keep in your room for now). After she gets used to this, you can try moving her bed into her own room.

If your situation includes your baby's father, you can also try having your partner be the one to rock the baby and settle her into bed. In this scenario, you should be in another room, so that the baby doesn't see or smell you. A variation on this that works for some people with enough space is for Dad and baby to sleep together, while you sleep in a different room. This accomplishes night weaning for some families with thriving older babies. When it feels right, you can get the baby to sleep on her own, and you and your partner can return to sleeping together.

Safety Information for Crib or Bassinet Sleeping

Here are some important safety tips for your baby when she is sleeping alone:

- The mattress should be firm and have a fitted sheet that can't come loose when your baby moves on it.

- Keep all soft bedding, pillows, and stuffed animals out of the crib.

- Look for a solid wood crib with a nontoxic finish (since your baby may start chewing on it someday).

- Make sure that the crib is well designed (especially if it is an old one), with bars that are too closely spaced for a baby to wedge her head between them.

- Don't allow any smoking in the room where your baby will be sleeping.

More About Mattresses for Babies and Adults

Choose mattresses carefully. Just a few decades ago, all mattresses were made of nontoxic materials, such as cotton, kapok, wool, straw, or feathers. People in many parts of the world sleep on grass or straw mats. Nowadays, most mattresses available contain materials made of formaldehyde, chemical fire-retardants, plastics, or petroleum-based chemicals. Some of these expensive, extremely comfortable mattresses emit toxic gases that make the adults who sleep on them feel sick. Obviously, no baby or child should sleep on such a mattress, especially in the tummy-down position. Some research that I find quite credible attributes much of the high risk of sudden infant death syndrome in Western countries to babies' reactions to the toxic nerve gases emitted by mattresses containing compounds of antimony, arsenic, or phosphorus.[1] This type of outgassing is bad enough, but it becomes worse when, after a few months of use, common household fungi get into the mattress, creating an even higher level of outgassing.[2] For this reason, it is wise to avoid using a mattress for your baby that has already been used by an older child, unless you wrap it in a thin polyethylene mattress cover. (This is a kind of plastic that doesn't outgas.) For more information, go to: www.preventcribdeath.com. Even a new mattress that smells like plastic should be wrapped in this kind of mattress cover as a safety precaution.

8

IF YOU HAVE A JOB OUTSIDE YOUR HOME

About sixty percent of U.S. mothers who have babies or young children are now employed outside their homes. No one knows how many of these children are nourished by their mothers' milk, but we do know that only about a quarter of U.S. employers reported having any kind of "lactation program" for their employees in 2007. The good news is that even if you need to return to your job just a few weeks after giving birth, it may be possible for you to coordinate it with nursing your baby. Many women mistakenly assume that it will be so difficult to continue nursing once their maternity leave is up that they either decide against nursing at all or give it up during the first week or so. I'm not saying that this transition is easy, but lots of moms who have outside jobs and are committed to breastfeeding have demonstrated that it can be done. The secret to success for many of these women lies in their planning and preparation while still pregnant. Hopefully, you will have at least six weeks after giving birth before you return to the workplace, as it sometimes takes about four weeks for your milk supply to become well established.

In order to keep breastfeeding after you return to work, you must gain some measure of cooperation from your boss. It's wise to draw up a written proposal, as putting your needs into written form will allow you to present all of the necessary facts without being interrupted.

What Should Be in the Proposal

Would you like to work part-time for a couple of months or do some of your work at your workplace and part of it from your home? If so, you will have to be the one to write up the new job description for yourself, defining where and how many hours you propose to work and outlining what your responsibilities will be. Be careful not to set yourself up for stress or failure by creating expectations that you may not be able to fulfill. Know, for instance, that you are not going to be able to do a full-time job in part-time hours. Be creative: If you are now working full-time and want to switch to part-time work, maybe you can find another employee who might job-share with you. If you want, you can build in to your proposal that there will be a trial period, after which you and your employer can assess how the arrangement is working out.

If there is no chance of transferring all or part of your paid work to your home, look for any available space at your workplace that might be converted with little expense into a lactation room. Take into account your employer's possible worries that your needs might be too expensive or complicated to accommodate, or offer easy ways for them to provide you with what you want and need. The following lists should give you some basic guidelines of what to ask for.

What You'll Need (at Least):

- Permission to pump at work.

- Break time during your workday.

- Privacy (a curtain, if not a door).

- A place to sit.

- An electrical outlet.

What You'd Like:

- A door with an inside lock.

- A sink with hot and cold running water.

- A refrigerator.

- A clean, pleasant room near your workstation.

- A comfortable chair, preferably one with arms.

- Flexible break time.

- A written policy that supports the right of nursing employees to pump in the workplace and forbids other employees from harassing or discriminating against nursing mothers.

A 2000 report found that seventy-five percent of women who participated in two corporate lactation-support programs nursed their babies for at least six months. If you work for a company that is among the seventy-five percent without a lactation support program, you should start writing your proposal early. Gather evidence on the benefits of such a program to both employer and employees, so you can present it to your employer. Many employers are simply unaware of the needs of mothers who nurse their babies, as well as of the benefits that come from the creation of an environment that facilitates workplace pumping. Your job, then, is to educate. Point out studies of existing workplace programs that provide appropriate support for lactating employees; these will demonstrate that such programs save employers money in increased productivity and decreased absenteeism because of illness.[1-2] Don't forget to mention a recent study that showed that if all four-month-old babies were fully breastfed, fifty-six percent of hospital admissions of babies this age would be avoided.[3] With numbers like these, you can point out that making it possible for more employees to breastfeed their babies is a good investment, one that is bound to lower the health-care costs borne by your employer.

Make sure that you are informed about your legal rights. Unfortunately, the United States still has no federal law to establish or protect a right to pump mother's milk in the workplace. However, legislation in this area continues to be passed, because of the activism of nursing mothers. Approximately one-third of the states have laws concerning employees' right to pump milk in the workplace, but these laws vary widely as to what they require of employers. Some—such as those in California, Connecticut, Hawaii, Illinois, Minnesota, Mississippi, Montana, New Mexico, New York, Oregon, Rhode Island, and Tennessee—require that an employer must allow pumping during breaks and/or provide a place to pump. Some other states use the word *may* instead of *shall* or *must* in their laws, which means there is no obligation on the part of the employer to provide what the law suggests would be nice. In any case, few states have laws providing for penalties for those companies that fail to follow the law; California, Hawaii, and Oregon are examples of states that do.

If you live in a state with a weak law regarding workplace pumping, keep in mind that even a law that doesn't require compliance can be helpful, because it establishes a guideline to employers as to what a nursing employee needs. For instance, if your state's law says that any space provided should not be a bathroom stall, that the space should be private or close to your work area, these provisions should be brought up in your negotiations with your employer.

Be aware of any other pregnant or lactating employees who might join in your quest for employer support for your pumping and storage needs—your employer might be less hesitant to help if you will not be the only person to benefit from a lactation program. It's worthwhile to find out if any of the mothers of older children who nursed them did secret pumping in a toilet stall. If so, these mothers might become useful allies.

Present your written proposal to the person at your company in the best position to provide the support you need. If you work at a fairly large company, there may be a human-resources department that is responsible for flexible work schedules, family leave, on-site day care, and family-friendly benefits. Keep in mind that many women, depending upon the job they have, are able to continue working as they pump, especially when they use a hands-free pumping bra. Given the right setup and a little practice, pumping can be combined with answering emails, making phone calls, or typing.

You can find some very useful resources on the Internet to help you with drafting your proposal to educate your employer. Look, for instance, at a United States Breastfeeding Committee report, "Workplace Breastfeeding Support."[4] You can find documentation there that ear infections, which keep mothers away from work on average one to two days per year, can be reduced by two-thirds to three-fourths by nursing the child or that an average of $400 per baby is saved for your employer over the first year. Look also at the pamphlet from "The Business Case for Breastfeeding, Steps for Creating a Breastfeeding Friendly Worksite: For Business Managers." It focuses on a company's potential return on investment in the areas of health insurance, absenteeism, productivity, and employee loyalty.[5]

Whatever your situation, even if you are the only employee at your workplace who is using a pumping station, please know that you are not alone. All over the country, there are women like yourself leaning toward their breast pumps, doing their best to get those last few drops bottled up. To combat your loneliness, it may help to join one of the online forums for pumping mothers. Try www.pumpingmoms.org, www.milkmemos.com, or www.workandpump.com. Checking out these sites while you are still pregnant will help you to better prepare for what is to come.

Returning to Your Job

I recommend that you plan, if possible, to return to work on a Wednesday or Thursday, rather than at the beginning of the week. This will give you the weekend to rework your plans, if you have a meltdown on your first day or two back on the job. Don't be surprised if you feel emotional as you approach the time when you must return to work. This is to be expected, as it is hard to anticipate how you are going to feel juggling your job, your breast pump, bottles, your child-care arrangements, and the reactions of your coworkers to your new status as lactating mother.

Some new mothers make the mistake of thinking that they should practice pumping and getting their babies used to drinking from a bottle before they return to work. I would advise against giving your baby a bottle during the first weeks after birth, because you will still be establishing your milk supply during this period. For most women, this means that your breasts will need as much stimulation as possible. Once your milk supply is well established at around four weeks, you can begin to try out your breast pump and to start storing some expressed milk in your freezer. It's a good idea to have about a week's supply of milk stashed there before you return to work.

Breast-Pump Basics

You will need to rent (hospital-grade pumps are rentable and designed to be safe for multiple users, unlike those designed for the consumer market) or buy a good breast pump if you have a job that you must resume while you are breastfeeding. You may need both a good electric model and a manual model if you are going to be traveling without your baby.

As mentioned above, electric breast pumps are considered to be single-user products, so it's better not to buy a used pump on eBay, share your pump with someone else, or sell yours when you finish using it. Milk can theoretically travel up the tubing and into the motor, which is impossible to clean. If your budget is too tight to consider buying what you think you need, check with your local WIC (Women, Infants, and Children) office, where they supply low-income women who are working or in school with pumps at a lower cost or sometimes free of charge.

"Loving Support Makes Breastfeeding Work" is the WIC breastfeeding-promotion campaign, which is national in scope and being implemented at the state-agency level. The goals of the campaign are to: encourage WIC participants to initiate and continue breastfeeding; increase referrals to WIC for breastfeeding support; increase general public acceptance and support of breastfeeding; and provide technical assistance to WIC state and local agency professionals in the promotion of breastfeeding. Visit the campaign's website at: http://www.fns.usda.gov/wic/Breastfeeding/lovingsupport.HTM.

You may not want to buy a pump until your breastfeeding gets off to a good start, as pumps are not returnable. Be sure to check out the facilities you'll have available for pumping before you decide which pump to buy.

Manual Pumps

Some manual pumps work by creating suction in a way similar to when the plunger of a syringe is pulled back on a vial of medication. These models feature a cylinder within another cylinder, with a rubber gasket sealing the space between them. The milk can be collected into the outer cylinder itself or into a separate bottle. Examples include the Kaneson Comfort Plus pump, the Lansinoh Easy Express, the cylinder hand breast pump, the Medela Spring Express or the Medela Manualectric, and the White River breast pump kit model 500.

Another type of manual pump is the hand-squeeze type. This kind allows you to squeeze the handle at the rate that works best for you, which may vary during a session (usually quickly in the beginning to stimulate letdown and then more slowly once your milk begins to flow). Examples include the Avent Isis, the Ameda one-hand breast pump, and the Medela Harmony.

Electric Pumps

The basic types of electric pumps are the battery-operated, the semi-automatic, and the fully automatic. Fully automatic or self-cycling electric pumps are generally the best choice for a woman who will be away from her baby for several hours a day on a regular basis or one who wants the machine to help build up her milk supply. The best models can be used to pump from both breasts simultaneously (cutting pumping time in half and increasing the amount of stimulation of your breasts). They also generate a suction and release pattern automatically, so you don't have to control this manually. The pumps that can provide forty to sixty such cycles per minute most closely mimic the sucking pattern of a nursing baby. These are the most expensive of the portable models, but they still cost about one-fourth to one-third of a year's worth of infant formula. You may find as much as a $100 difference between the top-grade model, which has a two-phase expression that mimics a nursing baby's rhythm and allows you to adjust the speed, and the next-grade model, which lacks both of these features.

The more expensive pumps allow for faster pumping (six to eight minutes) than the less fancy pumps (ten to twelve minutes). Examples of top-of-the-line pumps are any of the Medela Pump In Style line and the Ameda (Hollister) Purely Yours line (also marketed under the name Lansinoh) and the Avent Isis IQ Duo. Another pump in this category is Medela's newest Freestyle pump—a very small, battery-powered double pump that uses the newest computer-generated suck rhythms.

An inexpensive electric pump is not recommended, due to its weaker motor. It may be painful, since slow cycling tends to pull on tender breast tissue. Additionally, the slower speed will not give adequate stimulation to the breast, so your milk production is not likely to be impressive.

Automatic electric pumps often come with a battery-pack option and an adapter that plugs into the cigarette lighter of your car. When plugging

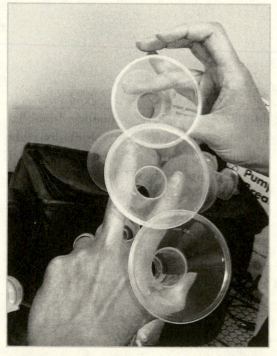

Breast-pump flanges

your pump into the wall socket, you will need a three-pronged outlet or plug adapter.

As a rule, it's better to buy a pump that has flanges made of soft silicone rather than a harder material. The advantage of buying a pump from either Medela or Ameda is that they offer additional sizes in their flanges, with larger nipple tunnels for women who need them. The average size is 24mm. The soft silicone petal massaging inserts further reduce that size. Approximately forty percent of mothers need a larger-sized flange to pump in comfort, due to either nipple size or breast elasticity.

The Basics of Pumping

Practicing good hygiene is very important in pumping and storing your milk. Dried milk left on your breast shields or any of your pump parts can be a medium for bacterial growth, which could infect you or your baby. Wash your hands with soap and hot water each time before handling the breast shields and the pump. You'll need to sterilize your pump or the pump collection kit before its first use if it is not already sterilized. The instruction manual that comes with your pump will explain what is necessary for your particular pump. You do not have to resterilize the pump parts, unless you are pumping for a baby in the NICU. If you are pumping multiple times in a day, studies have shown that, due to special live properties in human milk, it's not necessary to wash the parts of your pump each time. Once every eight to ten hours is sufficient. Washing your pump parts when you return home will save you time at work.

Learning how to pump effectively takes practice, just as nursing itself often does, so please don't give up if you don't get much milk into your collection bottle during the first few sessions. It may take weeks for you to learn how to effectively empty both breasts. It's useful for you to know that pumps collect only milk that you have let down. As you might guess from my earlier discussion of the letdown reflex, there are several things that you can do to help the right hormones reach sufficient levels for a good letdown and milk flow. First, make sure that you have a quiet, private place where you can pump comfortably. You'll tend to have more milk early in the morning than later in the day, so try to fit in a pumping session then. Do your best not to focus on how much milk is being released, since caring too much will actually inhibit the flow of milk—when you take your mind off being anxious about the quantity of milk you are releasing, your pituitary will be better able to release the oxytocin that will stimulate your letdown reflex. You may want to try some calming activities; for example, it may help to look at a photo of your baby, smell an item of his clothing, or even sit at your computer and visit a breastfeeding chat area, where you can communicate with someone else who is doing what you are doing. Breathe deeply and slowly as you pump. Rituals are important for many moms, such as pumping in the same place at the same time while listening to the same music. It can also be helpful if you massage both breasts before you begin. If you find that you're still having trouble stimulating your letdown, try leaning forward and using a comb to stroke your breast from chest to areola just before you pump. This tactic may sound odd, but it has worked well for some moms. You may also want to try applying a warm compress to your breast before pumping (though not if your breasts are engorged).

Most mothers need to pump for ten to fifteen minutes, with those last minutes achieving another letdown and resulting in the collection of extra milk. If you want to increase your milk supply, try massaging, then pumping for several minutes, massaging again, then pumping again. Remember that the more often you pump now, the more milk you will have later.

You must be well hydrated to do well at pumping. Make sure that you have plenty of water within reach while you are away from your baby and especially while you are pumping. One of the best ways to gauge whether you are drinking enough is to notice the color of your pee, which should be very light yellow.

Many women find that a hands-free bustier makes pumping far easier. Worn only while you are pumping, this bustier fits over your nursing bra. You lower the flaps of your nursing bra and insert the pumping attachments into the holes over the nipple. Once everything is in place, both of your hands are free for whatever you want to do with them. The Easy Expression Bustier is an example of this system. Medela also makes a hands-free kit that fastens any of their bras to their pumps' parts.

Pain While Pumping

Pumping your breasts should not be painful. If it is, it is important that you discontinue whatever practice is causing the pain, as this may be an indication that you are damaging your nipple or breast tissue. Even if this isn't the case, the pain will interfere with your ability to let down your milk.

One possible cause for discomfort is if you have a small pump that takes too long to generate a high enough suction before it releases the pressure (this causes discomfort for many women). Ideally, your pump should reach pressure after only a couple of seconds, then that pressure should be released. The suction levels should be high enough to get the milk flowing but no higher than that, as pressure that is too high for too long can damage your nipples. If you are having pain, try lowering the suction (which is sometimes labeled *vacuum*) until it is no longer painful. Please make sure that you don't confuse the suction setting with the speed setting if your pump has both features.

If pain persists after you have adjusted the suction, it may be that you don't have a good fit with the breast flange. Sometimes moistening the flange of your pump before you apply it to your breast may end your discomfort. Your breast should be centered within the flange, and your nipple should not be too large for it. If you have trouble seeing whether your nipple is centered within the flange, ask someone to help you. If that flange is too small, there may be friction right on your nipples, which will make them sore very quickly. Again, only Medela and Ameda make pump flanges with larger nipple tunnels for those women who need them. Keep in mind that your nipple may look wider to you when it is drawn into the tunnel.

Storing Milk

Your milk will keep for eight to ten hours at room temperature in a clean, covered container. You can store it in the coldest part of your refrigerator, where it will last three to five days, or in your freezer, where it will last up to six months. Your refrigerator door is the warmest part. Don't be surprised if your refrigerated milk separates. Try to gently swirl it to recombine it before use. Don't vigorously shake it, as this has been shown to damage the milk. Reheat frozen milk in a bowl of warm water. Never microwave it, as this destroys essential nutrients. After you thaw frozen milk, you should use it within twenty-four hours. You should not refreeze your milk.

It is best to freeze your milk in either glass bottles (being careful not to fill them too full, because frozen milk expands) or plastic bottles made especially for freezing milk. Ordinary resealable kitchen plastic bags are less durable, so it's hard to seal them once they are filled, and the seams sometimes burst when the bag is frozen. Besides, there are other problems with storing food intended for your baby in soft plastic bags, which I'll explain below.

Most working moms will need two sets of storage bottles: one to pump into that day and another, containing the previous day's milk, to take to child care.

The average woman makes between three and five ounces of milk per feeding, or thirty-two ounces or so per day. This amount doesn't increase over time—women don't need to produce gallons of milk, as cows do—because the number of calories per ounce in your breast milk will increase automatically to meet your growing baby's needs. And since breastfed babies are very efficient, their resting heart rates are lower than those of formula-fed babies, so they need fewer calories. This is one explanation for why breastfed babies have lower rates of adult obesity.

Soapy-, Metallic-, or Rancid-Tasting Milk That You Have Thawed

Many women find that their babies refuse to drink the thawed breast milk they pumped and froze days or weeks earlier. When the moms taste the milk themselves, they understand the reason: It has developed an unappetizing taste that mothers variously describe as soapy, metallic, rancid, or gross. The problem arises because the milk has an abundance of lipase, the enzyme that breaks down fat in the milk. If this is your first try at freezing and storing your milk and you are thinking of stockpiling as much as possible, it's a good idea to test-thaw some of your first batches of frozen milk to see if it has kept its good taste. It's no fun to throw away the milk you worked so hard to express. Test it weekly for a while, as lipase may continue to break down fats even in the freezer; this way you'll learn the "freezer longevity" of your milk (this varies from woman to woman).

There is a way to reduce the lipase in the milk that you intend to freeze, which can prevent your frozen milk from developing a nasty taste. Scald it just after pumping (the scalding point is when bubbles form around the edges of the pan before the milk reaches the boiling point). Next, cool it as quickly as possible and place it in bags or bottles in your freezer. Boiling the milk destroys some of its immune factors and nutrients, so be sure to take the milk off the heat before it boils.

It's better not to use a microwave for scalding your milk if you can figure out an alternative. Some women use a bottle warmer to scald their milk, whether at home or at work. They usually say that their milk tastes better when processed this way than when it's scalded on a stovetop. If you choose the bottle-warmer method, you should heat the milk to at least 145 degrees for one minute or 160 degrees for fifteen seconds (use a digital cooking thermometer to test). Next, put the bottles of scalded milk into a large container with ice water in it and, if possible, into the fridge at work. Once you are home, you can transfer the milk into the bags or bottles you'll use for freezer storage. A deep freezer works better for long-term storage than the freezer compartment in your refrigerator. Remember: If you decide to use glass bottles or canning jars placed in a pan of water for the heating process (in order to avoid heating plastic), be careful not to put the hot glass containers of your scalded milk into cold water right away. Doing so is likely to crack the glass. Let it sit at room temperature until it cools enough for you to be able to pick it up. Now it can be transferred into the containers that you'll put in your freezer.

Some women find that quicker thawing of the frozen milk makes for a better taste than thawing the milk in the fridge over a period of hours before use. If your thawed milk tastes bad to you but your baby doesn't reject it, don't worry. The high-lipase milk is not harmful to your baby.

A couple of other factors seem to affect some women's milk-storage problems. Omega-3 supplements, flaxseeds, and DHA supplements have all been reported to intensify the taste deterioration of frozen milk.

Buying Toxin-Free Products

We all know how convenient plastic can be when it comes to food storage. It's inexpensive, light, flexible, transparent, and durable. What many of us fail to realize is how unstable many plastic products are and how using them can introduce many unwanted chemicals, which may have adverse effects on health and normal development, into our bodies and those of our babies. This is a particularly important consideration for working mothers who will be bottling their milk.

One category of such chemicals, phthalates (pronounced "THAY-lates"), has been widely used in many of the products with which we come into contact on a daily basis. Phthalates are carcinogens that, when combined with polyvinyl chloride products (PVCs), form a flexible and durable kind of plastic that has been used to form countless consumer products. Phthalates can be found in plastic bibs, plastic wrap, plastic shower curtains, vinyl flooring, and countless plastic toys. They are also much used in medical equipment, including tubing and intravenous lines and bags. Until recently, they were present in most plastic pacifiers, nipples for baby bottles, and teething rings, and some of these products may still be available for purchase. (Please note: Don't buy used plastic pacifiers, nipples, or teething rings.) Phthalates are also found in some nonplastic products, such as shampoos, skin lotions, and detergents. A study published in 2005 by the Centers for Disease Control (CDC) found that seventy-five percent of the participants tested had detectable levels of phthalates in their bodies.[6] Those tested were all over the age of six, but all indications are that the levels of phthalates would have been even higher in babies.

The European Union started the debate on the toxicity of phthalates by passing a ban on the use of these chemicals in pacifiers, nipples, and teething rings in 1999. This came after advocacy groups such as Greenpeace began to publicize the results of animal studies revealing the adverse effects upon the male reproductive system. Such a ban has still not been passed in the United States, although some manufacturers now offer "PVC-free" pacifiers, teething rings, and toys on a voluntary basis.

Other health problems that have been linked to phthalate contamination include genital abnormalities in young males, premature breast development in girls, and poor brain and nervous-system development in both genders.

Many of us have become addicted to the toxic hard plastic products containing bisphenol A (BPA) used in baby bottles, other food containers, and the linings of food and beverage cans (including those containing infant formulas). BPA mimics estrogen in the body and seems to interfere with the bodily processes in which estrogen plays a key role. These include ovulation and reproduction.

When the advocacy organization Environment California tested five leading brands of baby bottles, it found that all five bottles leached BPA when they were subjected to the temperatures reached in most dishwashers. The levels of leached BPA were equal to those that caused harm in laboratory animals. Adverse effects included impaired sperm development, early onset of puberty in girls, higher rates of Down syndrome, impaired immune response, and higher rates of miscarriage. A 2003 study showed that even very low levels of BPA were associated with chromosomal abnormalities in laboratory animals. Don't believe the labels on plastic products stating that they are "microwave safe." An analysis carried out by the *Milwaukee Journal Sentinel* found that ten out of ten "microwave safe" plastic containers leached BPA.[7] Canada has declared BPA a toxin and has taken steps toward banning it from baby bottles, infant formula, and other children's products. The Food and Drug Administration, on the other hand, has declared it to be safe.

What to Use and What to Throw Away

Most plastic products have recycling codes printed on them. Often, there is a number inside the recycling logo.

Whether for babies or older members of the family, you can use codes 1, 2, 4, and 5 for storage (but never in a microwave or oven), and you should throw away any products with codes 3, 6, and 7. However, if you wish to lower your family's exposure to potentially toxic plastics, it would be wise to store all food in glass or ceramic containers.

Also, follow these simple points:

- Avoid sippy cups made of polycarbonate, because these can leach chemicals. Brands made from polypropylene or polyethylene are safer.

- Avoid Styrofoam. Insulated mugs with stainless-steel interiors are better.

- Avoid plastic wrap (it's polyvinyl chloride). Use waxed paper instead.

Don't forget that vinyl flooring often contains phthalates and that your crawling baby or toddler is likely to spend a lot of time on the floor. Look for flooring that doesn't contain chemicals that outgas (cork or hardwood flooring are good choices).[8]

Finding the right balance between a necessary, safe, and ecological use of technology while staying close to nature in all possible ways is one of the greatest challenges of being a mother in the twenty-first century. Every woman who manages to continue breastfeeding even though she has an outside job makes that path a little easier for those who come after her.

9

THE FIRST THREE MONTHS

Growth Spurt

During the first three months of your baby's life, it is quite normal for her to go through periods when she suddenly wants to nurse more often. At these times your breasts may feel emptier than usual after a feeding, and your baby may seem less satisfied after she finishes a nursing session. When she nurses at this increased rate for a period of three days or so, your milk supply will increase to match her need. It's not unusual for this to happen when she is at the following ages: two or three weeks, six to eight weeks, and three months. She is going through a growth spurt, and her behavior is her way of putting in the order for stepped-up milk production.

Slow Weight Gain

Make sure that you weigh your baby the same way every time—either naked or with a single dry diaper. Be aware that all scales are not calibrated to one another, so slight discrepancies are to be expected. If her weight gain is less than about six ounces per week during the first three or four months of life, or you aren't getting enough wet and poopy diapers per day, it's important to increase the amount of nourishment she is getting.

Why Isn't Your Baby Gaining Enough?

If your baby isn't gaining enough weight, and there isn't a problem with your milk supply or her latch, then her slow weight gain might have something to do with how you feel about nursing and whether or not you are comfortable with it. I have known women whose letdown reflex during the first several weeks functioned only when they were in a room alone with their babies, because they needed that degree of privacy. And I have known others who weren't able to let down their milk because they were confusing the pleasant feelings associated with nursing with sexual feelings. I first learned of this problem from a friend, whose first baby was gaining quite slowly, despite the supplemental feedings she was giving him in addition to nursing. As we discussed her feelings, she told me that nursing actually felt very good but that it seemed a little weird for her to be feeling that good with her infant son. My response was that nursing is *supposed* to feel good and that the pleasant feelings are what trigger the letdown reflex (and thus the release of the fat-rich hindmilk). Once she realized that what she was experiencing was normal, she relaxed and allowed the good feelings to flow. Her son began to get her hindmilk, and he started gaining well without further supplementation.

A similar case involved another friend who had nursed her first child, a daughter, for more than a year without a problem. Her next baby, a son, was born plump and healthy. When I noticed that his weight gain during the first month of life was poor, my friend asked me if I could pinpoint the cause. Her pediatrician had seen him and ordered lab tests, which came back normal. The doctor's recommendation was to begin supplementing with formula. As she sat with her baby on her lap with her shirt open, I saw right away that her milk supply wasn't the problem—milk was dripping from both breasts as we spoke. She told me that he sometimes seemed like he wanted to sleep more than he wanted to eat. Watching them together, I noticed that she treated him differently from the way she treated her daughter. With a concerned expression on her face, she held him a foot or so away from her body, looked at him intently, and asked him why he didn't want to nurse. Mind you, he was less than a month old. At that point, I suggested that she try smooching and cuddling him so I could see how he would react to some tender attention from her. When she kissed him on the cheek a couple of times, I saw an instant change in this skinny baby. He began to bloom, his eyes opened wider, and he began to relax his lower lip (which had been drawn in so far that it was barely visible). He responded so obviously to her treating him like her adorable baby boy that she couldn't miss her powerful effect on him. He rewarded her by gaining ten ounces that first week, and from that point on, he thrived.

Pacifiers can also be the culprit for a slow weight gain. Do you ever give your baby a pacifier? If so, put it away. Any sucking that she does should be on your breast. If not, the pacifier is getting the stimulation that should be telling your breasts to make more milk. Don't forget that night feedings are important for delivering the most milk during a nursing session to your baby.

Some babies with slow weight gain have trouble relaxing enough to take in the amount of milk that satiates them. They take a couple of swallows, then jerk away, sputter, get angry, and start to cry. If this happens with your baby, you may find it hard to get her to settle down long enough to get both the lower-fat and the high-fat milk from the breast. In these cases, after your initial letdown has taken place and your baby's nursing has slowed down, it sometimes helps to compress your breast to increase the flow again. Do this as long as it stimulates your baby to drink a little more from that breast. This may increase her intake on that feeding enough to get her really satisfied before she lets go and dives into deep sleep. Do finish off one breast before you move to the other.

Health Conditions or Illnesses That May Affect Milk Supply

Of course, it is also possible that your baby is not gaining properly because your milk supply is low, which may be caused by an illness or a physical condition. Is it possible that you are anemic? Anemia has been reported to contribute to low milk supply. If you lost a lot of blood during birth or if your hematocrit or hemoglobin was low before you gave birth, it may help you to eat more iron-rich foods, such as dark-green leafy vegetables, blackstrap molasses, unsulfured dried fruits, sunflower and pumpkin seeds, beets, red beans, and eggs. Seaweeds, especially kelp (also known as kombu) and dulse, are rich in iron and can be sprinkled in soups or on other foods. One to two tablespoons of seaweed flakes or powder can be taken per day. Egg yolks are also rich in iron.

Two diseases that can affect your ability to produce milk if they go untreated are underactive thyroid condition (hypothyroidism) and diabetes. Both diseases are diagnosed by blood test and are treatable. There are also several diseases or conditions that may be treated with medications that can decrease milk supply. These include depression, allergies, hypertension, migraine headaches, insomnia, and asthma. See Appendix A for information on the safety of various medications while breast-feeding.

If you have had postpartum bleeding that has persisted past six weeks, it is possible that a bit of placenta remains inside your uterus. This condition can decrease your milk supply in the early weeks. Check with your family physician or obstetrician if you think that you may have this condition.

Raynaud's Phenomenon and Nipple Pain

One rather obscure cause of nipple pain that might make nursing difficult during the first months of a baby's life is Raynaud's phenomenon. Though it is well known among physicians as a symptom of rheumatic diseases such as lupus, scleroderma, and rheumatoid arthritis (particularly when it affects the fingers), Raynaud's can occur in people who have no illness. It is generally triggered when there is a sudden drop in temperature or an emotional upset. The major symptom is that a couple of fingers turn white or blue and they hurt. When put into warm water, the usual skin color returns and the pain subsides.

Not many physicians are aware that Raynaud's phenomenon sometimes happens in the nipples of breastfeeding women. It doesn't usually occur while the baby is nursing but rather just after the baby lets go, when the nipple is exposed to the air temperature (which is cooler than the baby's mouth). A spasm in the blood vessels causes burning pain, and the nipple will become white or sometimes blue. When the spasm is past, the nipple will return to its normal color, and the pain may lessen or turn to throbbing rather than burning.

Raynaud's phenomenon is often associated with other causes of nipple pain, such as trauma from a poor latch or a thrush infection. When this happens, the treatment for the primary cause of the nipple pain will often solve the Raynaud's problem within a couple of weeks as well. Sometimes the application of heat alone will solve the problem, but other times it becomes necessary to try medication.

One medication you may want to try to eliminate pain from persistent Raynaud's phenomenon is nifedipine, a prescription drug that was formulated to dilate blood vessels in people with hypertension. The dosage in the case of Raynaud's phenomenon is one thirty-milligram tablet of the long-acting version of the drug. Take it for two weeks and then try to do without it. Very rarely, there is a case of Raynaud's that requires three or four two-week courses of nifedipine to achieve pain-free nursing.

Mona's story shows what a dramatic difference nifedipine can make to the lives of mothers with severe Raynaud's phenomenon that won't respond to home remedies.

❧ **Mona:** *Breastfeeding Ethan began to be challenging once we came home from the hospital. I had pain during feeding, but a few minutes after I was done feeding him, I would have this deep pain that, quite frankly, was awful. When I looked at my breasts at this point, the tips of the nipples were completely blanched. They were pale, almost white. This situation persisted for about a month, during which I obtained two different lactation consultations. Both checked his latch and our technique and confirmed that that was NOT the problem. They independently suggested that I may have Raynaud's phenomenon of the nipple. I could also elicit the pain if I went outside in the cool weather. I basically couldn't leave the house if there was the slightest breeze.*

I found brief periods of relief by taking hot showers and also by making socks filled with rice and heating them in the microwave. I would then put these in my nursing bra after nursing or to go outside.

A major breakthrough came when I heard about nifedipine, a vasodilator. I then made an appointment with my obstetrician and basically begged him to prescribe this for me. He was skeptical, but after researching the safety of the drug, he agreed that it would be safe to take it while I continued breastfeeding. He gave me enough for six weeks. I took one thirty-milligram tab each day for two weeks. My copy of Kathleen Huggins's The Nursing Mother's Companion *said only for the worst cases do you need to repeat this dose. After four to five days, I began to get relief. I was a completely different person and began to enjoy life again. Breastfeeding became a pleasure, instead of a painful experience. In my case, I stopped taking the medications after two weeks and the symptoms started to return. I immediately returned to the meds and took them for the full six weeks. I have had absolutely no pain since. Interestingly, when I went back to see my obstetrician for an annual exam, he told me that he has since had a few patients with my symptoms and has prescribed the nifedipine with success. He calls me his test case. My realization was that there is a disconnect between the lactation consultants who see nursing moms and the physicians. The lactation consultants had seen Raynaud's phenomenon many times in their careers, but the physicians had not. I am assuming this is because by the time the women who had experienced it made it to their six-week checkup with their obstetrician, they had given up breastfeeding because it was so uncomfortable.*

Before I was pregnant I used to jog a lot, and I would have some discomfort with my nipples if I stayed in a wet sports bra and it was cooler outside. I don't know if this is related.

Herbal Supplements to Increase Milk Supply

Several herbs are considered to be beneficial to supporting a good milk supply. These include alfalfa, raspberry leaf, borage, fennel, fenugreek, and blessed thistle. You may already have fenugreek on your spice shelf if you like to make Indian curries, as it is one of the principal ingredients used in this kind of cooking. You can take any of the herbs listed above in capsule form. I've heard the most positive feedback about the effects of fenugreek and blessed thistle used at the following dosage: three capsules of each herb taken three times a day. Another favorite of mine is six to eight alfalfa tablets per day.

One cautionary note about fenugreek is that this herb is a blood thinner. If your postbirth bleeding continues beyond five weeks and you are using fenugreek to increase your milk supply, it would be wise to stop using it until you stop bleeding.

Drugs That May Increase Milk Supply

Though there are quite a few prescription drugs that can be used to increase milk supply, several of them have serious side effects. Review the list below with caution.

- Several drugs that were originally intended for the treatment of schizophrenia can increase the release of prolactin by lowering dopamine levels in lactating women, thus increasing milk supply. The problem with these drugs, though, is that most—if not all of those available in the United States—have nasty side effects, such as tremors, uncontrollable twitching, and fatigue.

- Dr. Jack Newman recommends domperidone (Motilium) for increasing milk supply. Originally developed to treat gastrointestinal disorders, it is dispensed only with a physician's prescription. The Food and Drug Administration (FDA) warns against its use because of possible cardiac side effects (seen in sick mothers who were receiving the drug via intravenous lines). Be aware that this drug has not been tested in babies.

- Another medication used to increase milk production is Reglan (metoclopramide). It's said to be quite effective if used for a week or two, three times a day, in ten-milligram doses and then tapered off one dose per week. However, women with a history of depression shouldn't take it, as side effects such as weakness, fatigue, or depression can occur.

Using a Supplemental Nursing System (SNS)

Sometimes babies do need supplemental feedings. One way to deliver these without using a bottle (which can cause nipple confusion and interfere with your baby's sucking technique) is by using a supplemental nursing system (SNS) sometimes called a lactation aid. This is a small container—either a bottle or a plastic bag—that has a thin plastic tube leading from it to your breast. The tube should extend about a quarter inch past your nipple. The container is filled with expressed milk (or formula) so that when your baby suckles at your breast, she draws the milk through the tube at the same time that she stimulates your nipple, thereby encouraging more milk production. Some commercial models feature a container that can hang around your neck by a cord. Others have a clip that allows you to fasten the device to your clothing.

You can also fashion your own SNS by inserting thin tubing into a bottle, which you can set down next to you. You may have to experiment a little to find the right gauge of tubing to deliver a flow of milk that is neither too fast nor too slow for your baby. The tube must reach the bottom of the bottle without being bent.

Babies' Sometimes Inconvenient Preferences

Babies are like anyone else: If the milk flows more easily from one breast than the other, they may develop a preference for that breast. I have known a few babies who just refused to feed from one of their mothers' breasts. You will be comforted to know, though, that their mothers were able to nourish them quite well from the preferred breast. While you may feel somewhat lopsided, there is no real harm associated with one-breast feeding. Some women whose babies show this tendency learn to offer the least favorite breast first and then finish off with the "favorite" breast.

Some babies so prefer the breast to a bottle that they will refuse to take a bottle, even when it contains mother's milk. This can be a problem for you if you are a working mother. There's a nice little flexible plastic cup that works well for babies like these. It's called a Foley cup, named after its inventor (see Resources). Even very young babies can drink from this small, flexible cup, which can conform to the shape of your baby's lower lip. When introducing your baby to the cup, hold her propped in your lap at about a forty-five-degree angle. When she's calm and ready for a drink, give her a small amount of expressed milk and then wait for her to swallow before giving more.

Too Much Milk

If you are producing too much milk, and none of the tactics discussed on page 113 helped adjust your milk production, you might try to manually express some milk shortly before you anticipate your baby waking up. The removal of some of this foremilk can make it less likely that your baby has to cope with what must seem like trying to drink from Niagara Falls. It will also make it easier for her to get your hindmilk. Could you consider catching some of your overflow and making it available to a local milk bank? You will make someone else very happy by doing this.

"Colic," or Incessant Crying

All babies cry, but some cry a lot more than others. Babies who cry a lot during the early months of their lives are often called "colicky" or "high-needs" babies. They may spend many of their waking hours crying inconsolably, amazing you at their endurance and how directly their misery can impact your own inner peace. Young babies, especially those under the age of three months, cry for lots of reasons that may at first seem mysterious to you. They may cry from hunger, thirst, fright, because they want to be held, because they need to burp or fart, because they are uncomfortable, or because they don't like being wet or poopy. Sometimes they cry because they haven't figured out how to stop.

It's good to remember that "colic" is neither a disease nor a medical term. It's a grab-bag term that people apply to a baby who cries a lot. There are many things you can try to help your baby through a crying jag. As you go along, you'll get more proficient at understanding what's bothering her and what you can do about it.

Whatever action you take to calm your baby, you first need to calm yourself. If your baby's cries make you tense and nervous, you can relieve your own tension by slowing down your movements and deepening your breathing. Babies imitate their parents over the long haul, so be the kind of model you want your baby to copy. If you were a cat or dog, you would probably be licking her. I'm not saying that you have to do this yourself (although you may), but that's the kind of mood you should be in to calm your baby. Once you are calm, you will be ready to settle her down in whatever way feels most natural to you. For example, you might want to shush her, rock her, or gently pat her.

Crying sessions are often most intense between about four in the afternoon and seven or eight o'clock in the evening. If this is the time of day when you yourself feel the most tension, you can probably understand why your baby does too.

Don't be surprised if you get a lot of contradictory advice about how to calm your crying baby. Please don't listen to anyone who attempts to put you or your baby on a schedule. Clocks have nothing to do with this bond between breasts and babies. Time-honored ways of calming fussy babies include feeding, holding, rocking, swaddling, walking (outside when possible), singing, or making other soothing sounds. Do what you can to replicate the atmosphere of your womb—the rhythmic movement, the swooshing sounds, and the feeling of being held tightly.

Sometimes frequent crying in the first weeks of life is a matter of your baby's temperament. Extra-sensitive babies are more apt to show this behavior than babies of a more placid temperament. If you are the parent of a young baby who cries a lot, it's important for you to know that lots of very well-cared-for babies do this, especially during their first three months of life, and still turn out to be emotionally secure, good-natured people. If you are a first-time parent dealing with this, these months may seem like an eternity, but trust me, it will pass. By the time your baby approaches the age of three months, she will generally have gotten much better at calming herself. If not, you might want to have a look at Elizabeth Pantley's *The No-Cry Sleep Solution: Gentle Ways to Help Your Baby Sleep Through the Night.*

It could be that your young baby is crying so much because she is not getting enough loving touch from you. Like all newborn mammals, whatever their species, human babies tend to cry out when they are not in physical contact with their mothers or when they can't hear her voice or feel her presence nearby.

Sometimes the crying is closely related to feeding. If your baby is excited, almost frantic before a feeding, she may be breathing too fast to swallow without gulping down a lot of air with the milk when she is held to your breast. This will make her double up as if with stomach cramps and begin to scream. Sometimes it is possible to improve this pattern if you begin the feeding before she is completely awake and excited. Once she is already worked up, an upright position will help her burp, and some rocking and gentle swinging may calm her. Some babies nurse more efficiently in an upright position; in general, they swallow less air this way than when they drink while lying in your arms.

Wearing Your Baby

One of the first and most important technological innovations humans made tens of thousands of years ago were the cloth or leather baby slings that enabled mothers to have both of their hands free as they foraged for food. These slings are just as relevant today, as you'll likely find out if your little one requires your physical presence to stay calm while awake. Wearing your baby in a sling or baby carrier as you go about your day may greatly reduce the amount of time that your baby cries.

There are all kinds of slings available these days, and most allow several different ways for babies to be carried in them. Your baby may face you or face away from you in the sling. She may be snuggled into an upright position or a more horizontal position.

There are some safety tips related to baby-wearing that you should be aware of.

- Avoid standing at the stove or drinking hot drinks while you are wearing your baby. Eating, however, is all right.

- It's not a good idea to wear the baby sling in a car, as it is not meant to be a substitute for an approved car seat.

- If you drop something while wearing your baby, squat to pick it up instead of bending at your waist. Retrieve the dropped item with one hand as you steady your baby with your other. Bending at the waist is likely to cause strained back muscles, which can be painful for a long time.

You, During the First Three Months

Lack of Sleep

Waking up every two hours during the night can have a powerful effect on your consciousness. The struggle to wake up several times in one night when you have already been sleep-deprived for weeks can show you sides of your personality that you may not recognize. It may even cause you to do things during the night that you don't remember having done.

Here's a story about the mind-numbing fatigue of early parenthood, as told to me by my friend and fellow midwife Carol Leonard. As the single mother of a newborn son, Carol found herself more tired than she had ever remembered being. As her son's piercing cry rang out for the fifth time one night, her head throbbed with pain. Even though it was still pitch-black, she felt it would hurt her head less to feed her son with the lights off in her room. Opening her pajama shirt, she lifted her squalling son into her arms and held him to her breast. Instead of latching and settling down to eat, he writhed and thrashed in her arms and screamed even louder. Overwhelmed now, she burst into tears of frustration and self-pity as he wailed at maximum volume. Still unable to figure out what was wrong, she fumbled around in the dark and switched on the lamp on the bedside table. Now her problem was fully evident: She had taken hold of him upside down and was now trying to nurse his bottom! The absurdity of this situation, as well as the obvious solution, reactivated her sense of humor.

It's one thing to read a story such as this and another thing to experience the exhaustion that often goes with being a new parent. It's especially hard when you are the grown-up-in-charge more than ninety percent of the time. When you reach this level of sleep loss and fatigue, don't discount how helpful even a ten-minute nap can be. The same goes for how much of a boost you can feel when someone else holds your baby for ten or fifteen minutes. Avoid caffeine (which may make you more alert only in the short term), because your caffeinated milk may compound the lack-of-sleep problem by interfering with your baby's sleep patterns.

However tired you may feel from lack of sleep, you can always improve your physical and mental condition by relaxing. Take several deep breaths, making sure to exhale very slowly. Lower your shoulders and straighten your spine if you are in a twisted or slumped position.

When your baby has woken you up, avoid giving in to the impulse to hurry through a feeding so you can get back to sleep. If you move more slowly and deliberately, rather than rushing your baby, you will be less likely to make a mistake that will cost you your next nap.

Smile sometimes, even if you don't feel like it. It's times like these when you most need to smile. Maybe you will notice, as I have, that smiling when you feel rotten can lift your spirits. A smile has the power to instantly change your hormone balance within, which makes it worth doing. Hint: Even a sardonic smile can help. It's a step toward reactivating your precious sense of humor. Try to find a way to laugh at least once a day too—the more the better.

You may like singing to your baby. Music has the power to lift the spirits—both yours and hers. And it may also work for lulling you both to sleep. You should kiss her often and tell her how glad you are that she was born. She will get the message from your loving voice, and that should make both of you feel better.

Postpartum Depression

In her insightful *Of Woman Born* (1976), Adrienne Rich said it very eloquently: "My children cause me the most exquisite suffering of which I have any experience. It is the suffering of ambivalence: the murderous alternation between bitter resentment and raw-edged nerves, and blissful gratification and tenderness."

When a woman has postpartum depression, her experience dips more and more into the area of "bitter resentment and raw-edged nerves," and the moments of bliss and tenderness come fewer and farther between. Part of our problem is that doctors in the United States are taught not only that postpartum depression is prevalent—that between one and three million U.S. women will experience it every year—but that there is no way to prevent it. My own experience makes me disagree with this, because during my early years as a midwife, my partners and I used to comment on how rarely we saw postpartum depression among the first several hundred births in our community. When we did encounter a case, we could easily understand why the woman had postpartum depression, as she was invariably under some kind of extraordinary stress.

Here is a list of the many risk factors that are associated with postpartum depression:

- Sleep deprivation

- Poor nutrition

- Traumatic birth experience

- Fatigue

- Domestic problems

- Pain

- Prior history of depression

- Short (unpaid) maternity leave

- Stress over insufficient income

- High-needs baby, including preemies

- Sick baby

- Previously stressful life experiences

- Personality type that seeks to control

- Sore nipples and other breastfeeding problems

- Social isolation

- Unwanted pregnancy

The comparatively low incidence of postpartum depression in my community can be explained, I believe, by the good nutrition that all of the new women received, the rarity of traumatic birth experiences, the active intervention in cases of domestic problems, our system of flexible maternity leave, our tolerance for babies in many workplaces, and the absence of social isolation.

On the individual level, good planning during pregnancy can reduce your chances of falling into postpartum depression. If you and your partner are having domestic problems, for instance, it is important for you to seek help from a family therapist before the baby is born. You don't want the added stress of fighting with your partner when you are caring for a new baby at home, so it's better to get your problems resolved (one way or another) before your baby comes.

Social isolation is a major factor in many cases of postpartum depression. If you have no family members or friends living nearby, it's important to try to make some contacts while you are still pregnant. One way might be to attend a La Leche League meeting in your area. Befriending women from this or another breastfeeding group is a good idea, as they will be going through similar experiences and will be able to commiserate with you and help you with any problems you may have.

The nature of postpartum depression makes you retreat into yourself, feel that you are alone, and that there probably is no help for you. One of the most important things you can do if you think that you are sliding into depression is to ask for help. Here is a list of typical symptoms:

- Sad or anxious feelings

- Insomnia

- Headaches day after day

- Mood swings

- Poor appetite

- Ankle swelling

- Panic attacks

It is important to take active steps to address postpartum depression when you have these symptoms. Sleep and nutritious food are both restorative and can occasionally alleviate symptoms enough that no treatment is necessary. The help of a postpartum doula or a trusted family member or friend can also prevent the normal fatigue of new parenthood from progressing to postpartum depression.

You might also want to try making the following tea, which herbalist

Susun Weed recommends in her *Wise Woman Herbal for the Child-bearing Year*:

> *½ oz. chopped licorice root, 1 oz. raspberry leaf, 1 oz. chopped rosemary leaves, 1 oz. skullcap. Use 1 teaspoon of the chopped mixture to 1 cup of boiling water and drink 2 to 3 cups per day.*

Make a cup for yourself, or get someone to make one for you. Used in tandem with the other restorative measures discussed above, this tea will help soothe your frayed nerves.

Postpartum Psychosis

It is important to know that postpartum depression, if unaddressed, can worsen. Severe symptoms include:

- Violent fantasies
- Fear of hurting the baby
- Thoughts of suicide
- Hallucinations

Postpartum psychosis is much less common than postpartum depression, affecting about one to two women in every thousand. Like postpartum depression, it can occur as early as two or three weeks after birth, but I have seen it happen as late as seven or eight months following birth.

Fathers' Feelings

Fathers' feelings about breastfeeding matter a great deal. When a couple lives together, the woman will usually care very deeply about having the approval of her baby's father regarding breastfeeding. In fact, statistics have shown that if most men in a given sector of society decide that their wives shouldn't breastfeed, there won't be very much breastfeeding among the women of that social group. The opposite is also true—a father who is positive about breastfeeding can help his partner make breastfeeding work out well. For example, if a woman is extremely frustrated and is about to give up on breastfeeding because of some challenge—that may at the moment seem unsolvable to her but that could in fact quickly change—she may find that the true scope of the problem is put into perspective by an understanding spouse who values breastfeeding enough to help make it work. And if a woman doesn't have enough female relatives to give her the kind of support, ancestral wisdom, and practical knowledge that was traditionally shared among women when breastfeeding was the rule rather than the exception, a supportive partner can help compensate for that lack.

Helpful dads look for chances to change the baby's diapers and clothes, bathe or burp her, take her for a walk, sing to her, or comfort her. One of the major ways dads can help their partners with breastfeeding is by educating critical friends or relatives about the nutritional virtues of breastfeeding. Another important—and too often overlooked—way that a man can show support for his partner is to frequently let her know that her attractiveness is enhanced, not spoiled, by breastfeeding. Many women in our culture are uncertain about whether their changing bodies will continue to be attractive to their partners, so this type of reassurance will help give her the patience and persistence to get through the months ahead. I have met many wonderful men who are quite empathetic with their nursing wives or partners, and these guys are very creative in the ways they find to help their partners.

Both you and your partner will have to make many adjustments in the ways you relate to each other as you become used to being parents. Since your baby is the most helpless person in your family, she will become priority number one for you. And, since you will be having no lack of physical contact with her, you may find your libido dormant for the first few weeks of motherhood, as do many women whose libido was active throughout pregnancy. Your partner may not have anticipated feeling left out or rejected because of these changes. One of the most important things you and your partner can do during this stressful period is to make time together whenever you can, even though sexual contact is probably going to happen less frequently than before your baby came. Appreciate what he does to help you, and tell him how much it means to you that he doesn't complain when your share of the housework is left undone.

Your Sex Life

Several factors are likely to affect your sex life during the first few months following birth. These include the personality and needs of your baby, your birth experience, your own physical and emotional condition, your partner's work schedule, the number of older children you have, whether you have to return to a job, and your partner's needs. Add to these the sheer amount of attention that a new baby requires and the missed sleep and exhaustion that generally stem from this.

I recommend waiting until you have no more bleeding or discharge before you resume lovemaking that involves penetration. In most women, this process takes about three weeks. Waiting three or four weeks until the uterus is well closed protects you from infection during the postpartum period. Childbirth tradition from many cultures worldwide is that couples wait forty-two days before the resumption of lovemaking. Since we no longer have culturally agreed-upon norms, I think you are the one who should signal when you are ready to resume lovemaking—and you shouldn't feel pressured into it. If penetration hurts, you should wait, or choose some other form of loving your partner.

When you feel that you are ready, your lower postpartum estrogen levels may mean that you have a vaginal dryness you haven't experienced before. Natural lubricants such as coconut oil or cocoa butter may be helpful in this case. Another physical difference you might encounter while lactating is that if you have an orgasm while making love, you may spray milk. Keep an extra towel handy.

Breastfeeding as Birth Control

If you offer your breast whenever your baby is interested, day and night, your prolactin levels should be so high that you will be infertile for about six months following birth. Do you want numbers? You'll have less than a two percent chance of becoming pregnant as long as each of the following conditions is met:

- Your period has not returned.

- Your baby is drinking only your milk (with any supplemental feedings or drinks being given rarely if at all).

- Your baby is less than six months old.

- You feed your baby at least every four hours during the day and at least every six hours during the night.

As you can see, one of the advantages of night feedings is that they help suppress your return to fertility. Let's say that you have an outside job that involves regular separation from your baby. In this case, you'll need to express your milk at least as often as your baby would have nursed, with no more than a four-hour interval between pumping sessions.

10

AS YOUR BABY GETS OLDER

Pressure to Get Your Baby to Sleep All Night

It's a good idea to resist any pressure you receive from well-meaning friends or relatives to "train" your baby to sleep all night, especially if your baby's weight gain is less than it should be. Yes, sleeping all night is nice for you, but most nursing babies need to be fed at least twice (and maybe more) during the night throughout their first months of life. Lots of babies will continue to need that night feeding for several months. If your baby begins to sleep through the night and his weight gain slows down, it's good to increase the number of feedings during the day or to wake him during the night.

When trying to judge whether or not your baby is gaining enough weight, take into account that it's normal for babies who gained rapidly during the first few months to have a slower weight gain during the last half of the first year. Weight gain in breastfed babies between the fourth month and the end of the first year averages about four to five ounces per week. This means that the average breastfed baby weighs about two and a half times his birth weight at the age of one year.

As your baby grows older and more curious about the world around him, you may find that his weight gain slows down because he stops eating before he becomes full. Some babies nurse until they are stuffed, while others mess around and become distracted during a feeding. If you sense the latter is happening, you may find it more satisfactory to feed him in a quieter room with fewer distractions.

Teething

Teething ordinarily begins around the age of four to five months, and teething episodes may take place intermittently until a child is about two years old. A teething baby will usually drool more than usual and have tender, swollen gums in the places where a tooth is about to erupt. Most babies find teething uncomfortable to some degree. It can cause low-grade fevers, irritability, and fitful sleeping in some babies. If you've ever had a puppy, you know that teething time is when your shoes or slippers will be in danger, since all teething mammals want to chew on something; this is also true of babies.

There are several common remedies that can help the discomfort of teething in babies. Your initial response might be to gently massage the swollen gum in the area that is most tender. Most babies enjoy this (especially after the first few touches) and find it more comforting than chewing on their own fingers. You might also find that a chilled damp washcloth makes a great chew toy for your baby. Keep a couple of these in your freezer.

Many mothers have reported good success with homeopathic remedies for their teething babies: Chamomilla is one that is quite frequently helpful for babies who are extremely cranky and who like biting down hard on something. Babies are given the remedy in pill or drop form, and it helps relieve the urge to bite. Two other remedies that may prove helpful are Hyland's Teething Tablets, which combine a number of homeopathic remedies into little pills that can be placed under your baby's tongue at intervals to comfort his teething pain (visit 1–800Homeopathy.com to order), and Gentle Naturals Homeo-pathic Teething Liquid, which is made by Orajel.

There are also some over-the-counter medicines that you can find, but I would recommend that you try the ones mentioned above before resorting to anything that contains benzocaine, a numbing medication. This drug will numb not only the affected gum but also the tongue in that area, which can interfere with good nursing. Try to use a gel con-taining benzocaine only if your baby has trouble sleeping from teething pain and the more gentle homeopathic remedies don't seem to help.

You can give your baby anything to gnaw on that is not a choking risk (meaning that it won't break up into little pieces if your baby chews on it) and is not toxic. If you buy a plastic teething ring, make sure that you choose one that is labeled "PVS free" and "BPA free," since many of the teething rings still on the market may contain phthalates or BPA (Brio, First Years, Gerber, Haba, and Tiny Love are all non-phthalate products).

Biting

Babies, with extremely rare exceptions, are born without teeth, so biting is not something most mothers have to cope with during the early months of nursing. When babies begin to teethe, the tenderness and swelling of their gums often prompts them to clamp down on anything placed in their mouths, including Mother's nipple. Mothers who are taken by surprise will often give a loud yelp and immediately take the baby off the breast. Such a reaction is no more violent than any other mammalian mother might exhibit: It's quick and definite. It is normal for the baby to cry because of the suddenly interrupted access to Mother; more rarely, a very sensitive baby might be so startled by being abruptly set aside that he refuses the breast for a while. If you think your baby might be one of these sensitive ones, it might be a good idea to extract your nipple by inserting your fingers between his gums in-stead of removing him completely from your breast.

Nobody enjoys being bitten in a tender place, but depending upon how a mother responds to this, a bite can be a single or rare experience, or the baby can develop a habit of biting and the problem can continue (and worsen) for weeks or months. Occasionally, a mother will shy away from stopping the feeding when her baby bites, worried that her baby might start crying. She may even come up with a reason why his biting is her fault (maybe she let him drink from a kind of cup that required something like a bite), so she continues to allow it. When this happens, the baby eventually learns to enjoy hurting his mother, a situation that really does neither him nor her any good. In no other species would a mother allow this kind of behavior. When I encounter a situation like this, my advice to the mother is to study the behavior of other mammalian mothers by watching nature programs on television. Observing the mothering skills of other species can teach human mothers how to discourage certain behaviors in a firm way that is neither angry nor threatening.

I remember Amanda, whose response the first time she was bitten by her oldest child was an instinctive one: She let out a sharp cry. Her baby let go of the nipple and howled for a minute or two but never bit her again. However, Amanda told me that she felt so guilty about the incident that she wondered for months if she had permanently traumatized her daughter. It wasn't that her baby refused to nurse or seemed to be afraid of her in any way, but Amanda just couldn't forget that look of surprised betrayal on her baby's face once she let go of her mother's bitten nipple. Because of her guilty feelings, by the time Amanda had her second baby she had already decided that she would try as hard as she could not to follow her instinctual response to biting, because she could not fit it into her image of how a mother should act.

When her second baby was five months old and bit her sharply for the first time, Amanda took her off the breast and quietly but firmly told her, "No, don't do that. Don't do that. It hurts Mommy." Oblivious to verbal correction, baby number two kept on biting her. Frequent quiet lectures to the baby made no difference at all, and Amanda's nipples soon became so tender and sore that she ended up weaning the second baby much earlier than the first. Looking back on her two experiences with biting, she concluded that her instinctual response had actually been the better one, because it allowed the nursing relationship to continue longer. For what it's worth, both girls grew up to be sane, well-balanced adults.

Annie's story also shows how effective a mother's innate response to biting can be.

Annie: *My son already had some teeth, and one time he decided it was time to try them out on Mom and he bit me. I was not expecting this* *sudden attack and spontaneously pinched his cheek. (I did this without thinking.) He immediately let go of the breast and started crying. I pulled down my sweater and decided, "No more milk for him for a while." Then I noticed that he still had a red mark on his cute little cheek and I felt ashamed. But, still, you cannot have the baby you breastfeed bite you. The baby has to get a clear message of how to behave and how not to. I think that my response was almost like an animal instinct. At any rate, my son never bit me again, and so he kept on nursing for several more months.*

Tips on Keeping Biting from Becoming a Habit

It should not be necessary to wean your baby if he keeps wanting to bite you. Instead, your goal should be to teach him to continue nursing without injuring your nipples.

When your baby is teething, give him your full attention during a feeding. This way you'll be more likely to notice the mischievous look that usually precedes his bite. End the feeding if you see this look. It will often come after he has satisfied his hunger and has begun to get bored. I'm not saying that you can never read a book, talk to an older child, or talk on the phone while nursing your teething child, but it's not a good idea to do these extra things while you're teaching your baby not to bite you. Once the lesson is learned (which may take a few days), you should be able to return to a pleasant nursing relationship.

If your baby does bite, don't try to pull him from your breast when his gums or teeth are firmly clamped to your areola. Insert your finger between his gums or teeth, entering at the corner of his mouth, and then remove your breast. Be quick about it. After you've detached him from your breast, you should immediately and without anger set him on the floor (or several feet away from you). Don't resume feeding your baby for several minutes—although you can give him a cold washcloth or cold chew toy. How long should you wait before giving access to your breast again? Maybe ten to fifteen minutes; a minute or two usually isn't enough for the lesson to sink in. This doesn't mean that you shouldn't console him if he's crying; just don't offer your breast for a while. He won't starve, but he will get the message that biting causes him to temporarily lose access to the goodies. Contrary to what you may imagine, this will not break your child's spirit. It will keep your nipples from being damaged, which is important if you wish to continue nursing.

Punishing your baby's bad behavior isn't the only way to stop him from biting; you must also reward his good behavior. Don't forget to give praise or thanks when your baby *doesn't* bite you! The idea is to reinforce the behavior that you'd like to see.

Sometimes biting begins when Mother goes back to work. Usually, this kind of biting behavior changes when you give the baby your full attention while nursing.

Some mothers say that they can feel friction from the baby's teeth for a while during teething, even when the baby isn't biting. This friction may mean that the baby isn't latched as well as he could be. Take extra care to make sure that your baby's latch is good before going on with a feeding. The friction problem often solves itself when the baby learns how to hold his tongue in such a way to accommodate the new teeth.

Teaching Nursing Manners to Your Older Baby

If you never feel that you have become a martyr to your baby's needs, skip this section—it isn't for you. But if you notice, when your baby is around the age of seven or eight months (or older), that you have become a plaything for him in a way that doesn't feel good to you, read on. You may need to teach him some good nursing manners so that breastfeeding will once again be enjoyable for you, as well as for him. It's a good idea to teach manners as early as necessary, particularly if you want to continue nursing into toddlerhood.

Once a new mother's nipples have become accustomed to the baby's sucking and the baby has a good latch, nursing should become a sensuous and fulfilling experience for both the mother and the baby. It should not be a negative experience or an energy drain, even when Mother happens to be tired. Newborn babies, once they set up a regular sucking rhythm, melt onto their mothers, continuing to suck and rest until they are full or too sleepy to drink anymore. As the young baby grows older and friskier, though, he can become bored at the breast once his belly is full. When this happens, nursing may not be as comfortable and fun as it was when the baby was younger and more innocent. We're not talking here about the bite of a teething child who doesn't realize what he's doing; we're talking about the conscious actions of a bored child who decides to have fun playing with you, as if you were a toy. He may find it amusing to pull your hair or to tweak your other nipple while nursing or he may delight in kicking you with one foot while nursing. Maybe you don't mind this; some do, some don't. It is not really painful, but it is irritating. My recommendation is that you end the feeding just as soon as you sense that your baby has gone into this state of mind. Draw the line between feeding and playing. If your baby still seems hungry and ready to settle down for some serious eating, resume the feeding. If he moves again into irritating behavior, end the feeding again. Babies learn quickly if you are consistent. Another way to teach your baby nursing manners is to avoid feeding him when he's squirmy. Wait until he is in a calmer state of mind to begin a feeding.

You are not obliged to become a punching bag just because you are a mother. Allowing an older baby or toddler to punch, kick, or walk on you only teaches your child bad manners, which he will not only impose on you but perhaps on other people he meets later on in life. A mother who submits to abusive behavior from her own child runs the risk of raising a future adult who is inconsiderate of others. Linda described her son's antics this way:

Linda: *I enjoyed breastfeeding so much. I had plenty of milk, and my son grew and thrived. And thrived. And thrived. Pretty soon, he was a really big baby for a little old lady like me (I was forty-eight). He was a big, active baby who loved to play at the breast. He would pull on my nipples to look around, chew on them, and stretch them out as far as he could. I thought I knew all the tricks for training a baby to be nice, but this guy was really a workout. He was a wonderful child in many ways, but I began to suspect that maybe he wasn't the reincarnation of the Compassionate Buddha.*

I have known mothers who adopted such a submissive role in relation to their babies that they weren't able to enjoy them when they were three or four years old. It is easy enough to slip, step by step, into this position if you are already short on sleep and you have adopted the idea that you should always follow your baby's lead. It's important to realize that a young toddler who manages to dominate his (or her) own mother is hardly feeling secure in this role.

If your baby handles you in a way that isn't comfortable while nursing, you might try holding his hand firmly while he drinks. If he tries to pull away with your nipple in his mouth, release your nipple and set him off your lap. You may get a surprised or even a reproachful look. If so, remember why you did it. Mothers are not supposed to be treated roughly by their children any more than children are supposed to be abused by their parents. If the look is one of surprise, invite your baby to come back and finish nursing if you think he might still be hungry. If your baby doesn't learn what you want after one interaction such as this, repeat it as necessary.

Breast Refusal in Older Babies

Babies who have been successfully nursing for weeks or months sometimes refuse the breast. Although this behavior is not common, it can be upsetting. It's a good idea to calmly assess how much of a problem really exists. Older babies might refuse the breast during the day but nurse as well as ever during the night—enough so that they continue to gain well. If your baby refuses the breast sometimes but still feeds well three or four times per day, he will probably be taking in enough milk to remain healthy. You should make sure that your baby isn't becoming dehydrated, though, by counting the number of wet diapers you get per day (six in twenty-four hours should be enough).

Trying to force your baby to nurse when he doesn't want to tends to aggravate the problem. Gentle coaxing may persuade him to return to the breast, particularly if he's sleepy, or you can try to express some milk and see if he'll take it from a cup. Remember that a sleepy baby will usually be more likely to nurse.

Though it is rare, there are some medical reasons why a baby who previously nursed eagerly might refuse the breast. For instance, a baby with an ear infection might refuse to take one of your breasts if he would have to lie on his infected ear in order to reach it. The same goes for a baby whose nose is congested because of a cold. In either case, changing your nursing position might solve the problem—for example, you may do better if you feed him in a more upright position than usual. If he is still unwilling to nurse, he will probably drink your expressed milk from a cup. Try using a cool-mist vaporizer in the room where he will be most of the time, as this can help address the underlying problems. Many short feedings may work better than fewer long sessions.

Your baby might also be refusing your breast if you have mastitis or a blocked duct, since these conditions can create congestion in your areola or a portion of your breast that slows down the flow of your milk. You will need to remedy these problems as soon as you suspect them, as both can lead to more-serious conditions (see pages 131 through 136).

There are a few other possibilities to explore when your once-eager nurser refuses the breast:

- Sometimes the problem may be that you have given him too many bottle feeds or solid foods at too early an age.

- Anything that is emotionally upsetting to you can affect your baby's nursing patterns as well.

- If you have a knot in your midsection because of family tension, your baby may reflect this by temporarily refusing to nurse.

Concentrate on getting your milk into your baby, and avoid other drinks, such as water, juice, or formula. See pages 113 through 117 for more possible explanations for breast refusal. Whatever tactic you take, you should carry him around with you, getting as much skin-to-skin contact as possible, because this cuddling attention and proximity to your breasts may entice him to nurse. Most babies will pass through this phase and return to their former nursing patterns, and you may never know what prompted his refusal to nurse.

Effect of Birth-Control Methods on Feeding

Sometimes babies become fussy at the breast because their mothers have begun to take birth-control pills containing small amounts of estrogen. Even low levels of estrogen can decrease some mothers' milk supply significantly. This is likely to be part of the reason for your baby's trouble if he was gaining well and contentedly nursing for several weeks and then became fussy within a week or so of your going on the pill. Another indication that this is the problem is if your baby seems to want the breast but then pulls away, frustrated, after he starts nursing. By doing this, he is showing you that he is hungry but that the slow flow of milk is unsatisfactory for him. The best remedy for this problem is to stop taking the pill.

There are two types of intrauterine devices (IUDs) available in the United States today: One, the Mirena, releases small amounts of progestin, which causes the uterine lining to thin too much to support implantation. Because the Mirena does not release estrogen, it is supposed to have no negative effect on milk production. The American Academy of Pediatrics considers this contraceptive method to be compatible with nursing; however, while many women do not experience any noticeable reduction in milk production, I have heard of at least one case in which a mother's milk supply did drop significantly shortly after this IUD was put in place. That one case may have been an anomaly. Women who easily forget to take the pill and don't like barrier methods tend to be happy with this device. Some women have reported lighter periods once the Mirena was in place for a while, and others have said that it caused them to get more yeast infections than usual.

The other IUD available in the United States is the ParaGard, a copper variety that is completely nonhormonal (the metal seems to have a spermicidal effect). Some women find that this IUD causes longer and heavier-than-usual periods.

IUDs are not considered advisable for women who haven't already given birth, because the smaller size of the uterus makes for more irritation and a higher rate of expulsion of the device. Additionally, they aren't a good choice for women who will have more than one sex partner, because of the risk of infection.

Starting Solids

Many babies are ready to eat their first solid foods at about the age of six months. By this time, your baby will probably be able to sit up, pick up food, and put it in his own mouth. There are several good reasons to delay offering solid foods until the six-month mark. Exclusive breastfeeding provides your baby with immunities to many ailments during his most vulnerable period and protects him from many childhood diseases; also, babies less than six months old who are nursing well will get all of the nutrients they need from mother's milk. Since their digestive systems haven't matured sufficiently to digest foods other than your milk, there's no reason to introduce solid foods before this time. Poorly digested solid foods are a burden to the baby's system, which may lead to stomach pains and uncontrollable crying. It is especially important to delay this introduction if you have family members with allergies. There is supported evidence that food allergies, asthma, and runny noses have been linked to early introduction of solid foods.

Once your baby has begun to show signs of interest in what others are eating and is about six months old, you might want to experiment with introducing a new food. Some babies may not have any interest in solid foods even at the age of eight or nine months of age. If this is the case with your baby and your doctor is concerned, you can get your baby's iron levels checked with a simple hemoglobin test. Breastfed babies absorb the iron they get from mother's milk with great efficiency, so it's rare for breastfed babies to become anemic.

It's a good idea to nurse your baby before you first offer him a solid food. Introduce only a single kind of food at a time, as this will help you pinpoint whether he exhibits sensitivity to it.

Watch him closely for allergic symptoms. These include:

- Rashes or a sore bottom
- Gas, vomiting, diarrhea, constipation
- Nasal congestion
- Ear infection
- Fussiness
- Asthma or wheezing

If he likes what you have introduced and he doesn't react badly to it, continue supplementing his diet with only that food for a few days before introducing another. Avoid the temptation to give him as much as he will accept; it's better to start small until you see how he tolerates each addition to his diet.

Foods to Offer

Some good choices for your baby's first food include avocados, potatoes, mashed bananas, or sweet potatoes. Most babies like these foods, they are unlikely to cause allergic reactions, and they are easy to prepare. Watch your baby closely to see if he is able to swallow, without choking, whatever you offer him. Take your time and be patient.

Foods to Avoid

It's a good idea to avoid offering dairy products during your baby's first year of life. Many people are allergic to cow's milk, and your baby will not be missing out on any essential nutrients if you don't feed him dairy products. Eggs, peanuts, citrus fruits, strawberries, and raspberries are other foods that should be withheld during the first year of life, since many young children are allergic to them. You should also avoid feeding your baby foods that are fried or high in saturated fat, those that are quite sweet, and those that are flavored with artificial flavors or sweeteners. Salty crackers and potato chips are two examples. Not only do these types of foods contain unhealthy additives, but they will also overstimulate your baby's tender taste buds. Honey should also be avoided, as it may contain botulism spores that his immature digestive system cannot handle.

If you choose to offer your baby raw vegetables, you must grate them very finely because of the danger that he might choke on too large a chunk. If pieces come through undigested in his diaper, it's a sure sign that this food did him no good at all. Steamed vegetables that have been run through a food mill will be more digestible and will still be nutritious.

11

NURSING TWINS . . . AND MORE

Nowadays, many people seem to think that having twins is no big deal—we keep hearing about people who are having three, four, or even more babies from one pregnancy with assisted reproductive technologies. People who underestimate the difficulty of having twice as many babies as usual often haven't raised twins themselves. Having twins and more *is* a big deal; it requires new mothers to care for more than one helpless infant at once. Add to this the fact that multiples are more likely to be born prematurely, at low birth weights, and are more likely to need extended hospital care. For these reasons, you may have a rocky start with breastfeeding; you could find yourself caring for two or more hospitalized babies.

It's a good idea to look for a support group for mothers of multiples in your area while you are still pregnant. Listening to the stories of those who have traversed this territory before you will help you prepare better for what is ahead. In case there is no such group near you, try visiting an Internet forum for the mothers of multiples. Your morale will benefit from hearing the stories of other mothers who have managed to breastfeed their twins or multiples, and you will also pick up some useful tips on caring for your babies.

Lots of women can produce enough milk to feed two babies. For you to increase your chances of joining this lucky group, do your best to eliminate any other sources of stress from your life. Realize that you will need plenty of help during the first weeks and months of your babies' lives, whether or not they are born prematurely. Accept any help that is offered and ask your relatives and friends for more if necessary.

If you plan to give birth in a hospital, find out if there is a lactation consultant on duty at all times. Having the help of a professional lactation consultant will increase the chances that your babies will latch correctly in the beginning. This can do much to prevent later problems. Remember, a woman with only one baby can have trouble getting that baby to latch on right, especially if she is physically exhausted, sore, or left to her own devices. Having two babies to cope with instead of one isn't going to make things easier. Think of each baby's need for eight to twelve feedings a day once your milk is fully in and then multiply that by the number of babies you expect. At the same time, realize that thousands of women out there will testify that the rewards are well worth the trouble and persistence attendant to nursing multiples. Approach the challenge of feeding your babies one day at a time.

Find out if postpartum home visits after hospital discharge are part of the maternity-care plan you have. If they're not, start making plans while you are still pregnant about who (besides your partner, who will also be sleep-deprived) can help you during the first month or two.

Claudia's story shows how much the support of family and friends can help when caring for and nursing multiples. She faced a surprising challenge when she gave birth to triplets after expecting only twins. Fortunately, and unusually for triplets, her babies were full-term at birth. Here is her story:

✤ **Claudia:** *My labor was quick. I cannot say that I was in pain. I just felt uncomfortable. When my midwife arrived, I had been in labor for an hour and a half and was already seven centimeters dilated. It was a fantastic labor and delivery. We had a roomful of people, but in the end we didn't really have a surplus of people, because so many babies came out. Remarkably, each baby weighed nearly seven pounds.*

I decided to breastfeed all three. That went really well, mainly because

I had good people around me who were supportive of my decision. There was never any question that I would do it another way. Nobody treated me like I was crazy for trying to breastfeed all of them. My friend, my father, and my mother came, and while I breastfed one of the babies, they would cuddle and care for the other two. I had somebody with me most of the first three months. It was hectic. Usually it was me and at least one other adult, which was minimal, and the three babies.

But I got so much strength from doing that birth the way I wanted (I gave birth vaginally) that it carried me through the hard times of that first six or seven months. We'd be so exhausted by evening, and we'd have to take a deep breath, knowing that we would have to get up in the middle of the night with them. But we did it.

If you have a cesarean, keep in mind that it's still possible for you to nurse your babies—and doing so will yield real benefits for you and your babies. You will need help from a lactation consultant while you are in the hospital, and you'll definitely need help once you are settled back in your home after your discharge. If your babies are still hospitalized when you are released, try to have a family member or friend (besides your partner) come to the hospital with you and be with you as you nurse your babies. It is not unusual in cases of multiple births for babies of the same mother to be discharged at different times. In this difficult situation, you'll need a lot of help to manage the logistics of maintaining your connection with both babies. Again, a supportive friend or a relative will prove invaluable to you. In this case, you'll almost certainly need a heavy-duty breast pump, so you can nurse the home twin at one breast while pumping the other breast to get milk for your hospitalized baby.

Nursing for Two

While you are pregnant, you should buy a large U-shaped foam pillow, with a removable cover, that will wrap around you. The best variety has a strap that fastens behind you and an upper side that is angled so your babies are held close to you with their heads in the best position for swallowing. See Resources for more information on buying one of these. With such a pillow, you may be able to feed your twins simultaneously.

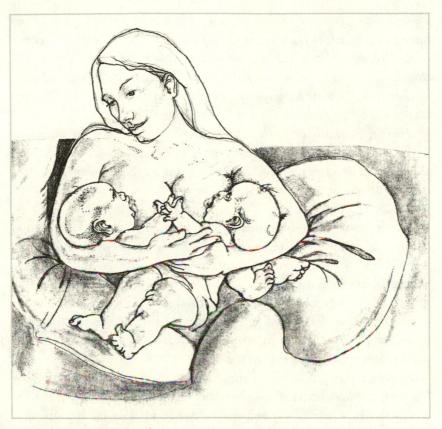
Simultaneous nursing with twins

However, in many cases, each baby will need to have developed a good latch and be able to nurse well before you try simultaneous feeding. Getting your twins to feed simultaneously probably won't be easy the first few times you try it, but it should get easier with practice.

Cara, a first-time mother of twins born at full term, wrote about her feelings the first time she tried nursing both girls at once:

Cara: *All went well until they both began rooting and crying at the same time. I tried nursing one at a time but couldn't stand watching my other girl turn beet red and scream at the top of her lungs. It was making my head pound fast into a throbbing headache—I was a wreck, and I started to cry too. How was I going to do this? What was I going to do? Get it together! After a couple of deep breaths, I arranged all the pillows that were around me, so that each pillow would support one of my girls.*

I decided to go for the underarm hold, which meant placing one of my hands under each of their necks for support, with their heads under my breast, ready to latch on. It took a while; they were worked up and thrashing around, and it was hard to get them on the pillows. Once I latched one, I'd have to reach up and try to latch on the other. The first would fall off by the time I got the second one on.

Finally, we made it! Both babies were happily latched on and nursing. At this time the new shift nurse came in. She was quite pleased, and we appeared deceptively calm. She brought me a breastfeeding pillow for use next time—just what I needed.

Simultaneous feeding stimulates both breasts at once, which is good for increasing milk production to meet the needs of your two babies. Even if one of your babies isn't as efficient a feeder as the other, the more efficient twin may help to facilitate a good letdown, thus benefiting the less expert feeder. In this case, though, it's a good idea to alternate breasts with each feeding, so that your breasts are stimulated as equally as possible. This will make it less likely that one of your breasts will be significantly larger than the other.

However nice and efficient simultaneous feeding sounds, some babies simply nurse better when given their mother's undivided attention. It will also be easier to know if one baby has an early latch problem if you feed them separately. (Sore, misshapen nipples will be a tip-off that at least one twin is having a latch problem.) If you have sore nipples, I recommend that you feed your babies separately for a while, even though it may seem at first that this will take more of your precious time. You may find that, by feeding them separately, you are better able to teach each baby the best possible latch, which will mean a better letdown of your hindmilk and better-satisfied babies.

Keep in mind that there is no one right way to feed twins. You won't know what works best for you until you get started. It will help you to figure out if you are meeting both of your babies' needs if you make a chart to keep track of how many wet and poopy diapers you get from each baby over the first few weeks. It's a good idea to continue this practice until you are sure that both babies are gaining weight at a good rate. (Hint: Prepare the chart while you are still pregnant.)

If your babies don't nurse well simultaneously, you might want to devise a system for keeping track of which baby you nursed last during the night. Sometimes a mother of twins may wake so many times during the night that she can't trust her memory about which one she most recently fed.

Quite a few mothers of twins are happy to own a heavy-duty electric double pump that will allow both breasts to express milk simultaneously. Some of the models that work with maximum efficiency are the Avent Isis IQ Duo, the Ameda Egnell Elite, the Medela Pump In Style, or the Medela Lactina. See Chapter 8 for more details on breast pumps.

Positions for Simultaneous Nursing

You may want to practice these positions with dolls or teddy bears while you are still pregnant. Have plenty of water for yourself within reach.

Double Underarm Hold

Putting both babies in the underarm hold works for many mothers. You may need a pillow or two behind you at the same time that each baby is supported on your twin-sized U-shaped pillow.

Double Cuddle or Cradle Hold

In this hold, both babies are cradled "crisscrossed" to your breasts, with their legs underneath each of your arms.

One Underarm and One Cuddle

One baby is positioned under one of your arms, while the other is cradled to your breast.

Supplemental Feeding

Sometimes supplemental feeding is necessary with twins, particularly immediately after birth. Tamara, a first-time mother of twins, had her babies vaginally at 37.5 weeks' gestation. Her babies were given formula during the early days because her milk was slow in coming in. Tamara soon learned how much difference a bottle can make during these early days. She wrote:

❧ **Tamara:** *Not all bottles are equal. Nipples come in a variety of sizes. You want a nipple with a wide base, as latching on to a wide-based nipple is closer to latching on to a breast and helps babies maintain a good latch while your milk supply builds up. Sasha didn't have jaundice and was better at getting colostrum from me than Cormac was, so for Sasha we used an Avent bottle. Avent bottles are especially designed to help babies maintain a good latch. I do believe the difference in bottles was a factor in Sasha maintaining a good latch and Cormac totally losing interest in breastfeeding by the end of the first week.*

While in the hospital, Tamara was encouraged to pump every few hours and received several consultations from her obstetrician, her labor doula, and others. She wrote:

Oddly, all this support made me feel like a failure. I could not get more than a few drops of colostrum from the pump—not even a teaspoon after twenty minutes of pumping. I was incredibly sore from the pump and trying to nurse two babies—I even got blisters. I would sit at the pump, crying, thinking of all my friends who had had no problems with breastfeeding and of one of my little babies who so badly needed the breast milk. Things changed quite a bit when we got home from the hospital and were greeted by my postpartum doula. She immediately pointed out that the flanges for my pump were too small, a big factor in the blistered nipples. [Too bad this problem hadn't been noticed days earlier.] She also advised me to rub the flanges with olive oil, which made a huge difference, and had me cover my breasts with ice packs after each pumping session. More than that, it was her positive attitude that helped. She'd known plenty of women who had to pump for a week or two, and plenty more who had to supplement. She assured me that the tiny drops of colostrum I was able to provide for my babies were doing their job and helped me make an appointment with another lactation consultant.

My postpartum doula also pointed out, on day three after coming home from the hospital, that I had mastitis. I was feeling terrible, had a fever, and my left breast was incredibly sore and hot. I'd assumed this was what I was supposed to feel like. I would have become extremely ill if it weren't for my postpartum doula. New mothers don't necessarily know how to diagnose problems like this.

Cormac had a very powerful latch too, but he was hungry and extremely impatient. He wanted his milk! After a few days of trying to nurse, he gave up on nursing and insisted on the bottle. How do you deal with a baby who rejects your breast? Many women throw out the bottle and force them back on. But if your milk isn't there and your babies are small, you don't have that luxury. I continued to offer Sasha the breast throughout the day and would offer the breast to Cormac a couple of times each day. He finally took to the breast after a bath. It was his first bath, and I think it took him back to the womb. After that, I noticed he was willing to nurse if it was late at night or early in the morning, when he was in more of a sleep state. At six weeks I finally had a good milk supply. But by then my son would cry and push me away when I offered him the breast—unless it was in the middle of the night.

I'm sure that using a lactation aid would have helped with Cormac, and I did buy one. But I was too tired and overwhelmed with everything (not just breastfeeding) to want to deal with this contraption in addition to everything else. And, to be totally honest, I needed to be able to hand a baby off to a helper so I could have a break. I therefore focused my breastfeeding sessions on Sasha during the day and Cormac at night, when he was more willing. Also, I would always breastfeed first and then supplement with the bottle.

It helped me to learn through online chats with members of a multiples group that my challenges were the norm. They also commended me on my perseverance. Many parents said they quit after a few weeks and felt much happier, as they could then focus on all the other aspects of being good parents. Even those who had successfully breastfed from the get-go were sympathetic and supportive about my need to supplement.

Getting Sleep

One of the hardest parts of being the parent of twins or other multiples during the first year is how much you'll yearn for more sleep. You'll want to get your babies to sleep at the same time as each other—so that you can sleep then as well—but getting there will take patience and persistence on your part. There is no one strategy that will work for everyone, and much depends upon the personalities of you and your babies. One way to encourage this sleep pattern is to try putting both babies to sleep in body contact with each other, as many twins have a way of calming when they are in contact. This can be done whether you are co-sleeping or if you put your twins in a crib together. If you find it possible to feed your babies simultaneously, you may want to wake one twin whenever the other wakes so they'll be on the same eating schedule. Then you can all get some sleep at the same time between feedings. Since most mothers find that feeding twins simultaneously requires sitting up, you'll want to do what you can to teach your babies to be awake more during the daytime hours than at night. Since newborns are usually on a reversed sleep schedule, you shouldn't expect them to immediately fall in line with your plan. It's hard enough to get one baby to do this, let alone two. To change this, you may have to make an extra effort to play with and excite them during the day, keeping the room they're in well lit. At night, be sure to keep the lights off or dim them as you tend to your babies' needs.

Babies who once nursed well together may interfere with each other's nursing when they're older, by interacting enough to be distracting during a feeding. Some mothers find that everyone gets more rest if the babies sleep on either side of Mom, who turns from side to side to feed each. You'll probably need a king-sized bed for this, and you might want to put the mattress on the floor. Even though this arrangement will probably mean several wake-ups during the night, you will eventually learn to nap as you nurse the babies. There are also mothers who like to leave the room with the baby they're feeding so they don't wake the second baby.

Many mothers find that they have one calm twin and one who is needier. While you may feel compelled to pay more attention to the one who's needier, don't forget to give your calm baby plenty of loving attention too. In this situation, it may be a good idea to swaddle the needy twin (or both of them) during the night, making sure that the covers over them (and you) can't accidentally be pulled over their faces. Swaddled babies can, of course, be placed side by side.

Nursing While Pregnant

One morning, years ago, my seven-month-old son abruptly refused to nurse anymore. He had seemed hungry and eager to nurse, but as soon as he tasted my milk, he pulled away, as if it didn't taste the way he expected it to taste. I soon realized that the reason for his behavior was that I had become pregnant. Apparently the flavor of my milk had changed in a way that was not palatable to him. Fortunately, he was good at drinking from a cup by that time, and he was able to make a smooth transition to other foods that agreed with him.

Many mothers become pregnant while they are still nursing a baby. For those whose babies don't wean themselves, as my son did, the question often becomes whether to wean or to continue nursing while pregnant.

In order to make this decision, there are several things you should know:

- It's not unusual to experience some nipple soreness when you are nursing while pregnant. This can either be caused by the hormonal changes that come with a new pregnancy or by a diminished milk supply, which may be triggering your baby to suck harder at your breasts to stimulate more output.

- As long as you are eating well, you needn't worry that your continued milk production will damage your unborn baby in any way.

- Don't worry that uterine contractions, which can be stimulated by nursing, will tip you into premature labor. (However, if you have a tendency to go into premature labor, and you worry about another premature birth, it would probably be a good idea to go ahead with weaning.)

If your new pregnancy turns out to be a difficult one, though, I would advise that you wean. How do you feel when you nurse during early pregnancy? Do you dread a nursing session because you are nauseous or more fatigued than you were before conceiving? Do you feel irritable? Most mammals probably would wean, given such signals from the body. But this is a decision that's up to you. You may have some strong reasons for wanting to continue nursing your older baby while your new one develops inside. Try not to have too many preconceived ideas, and take it one day at a time.

Tandem Nursing

Let's say that you've decided not to wean your older baby and to go on with what is popularly called "tandem nursing." When your new baby is born, your milk will switch to colostrum, ready for your new baby's arrival. From this time forward, your new baby must be given first priority at your breast. You may notice that your older child is affected by the laxative effect of colostrum if she nurses from you during the first two days after her sibling's birth. Looser, more frequent poop is common in such a case.

If you decide that tandem nursing is the best choice for you and your children, you are the one who is in the best position to decide whether it makes more sense for you to feed them both at once or separately. It's important for you not to feel bullied by your older child. You may need the support of other family members or friends to deal with any conflict that arises if your older child becomes jealous or wants to nurse whenever the new baby needs to.

You may have talked to many women who loved nursing their older children during pregnancy and beyond and have no regrets about their decision to go on with it. Others continue nursing because it seems the gentlest way to deal with their older child, who was not a self-weaner. Yet others find that the reality for them is less pleasant than they thought it would be. Gradual, gentle weaning may turn out to be the best course in such a situation. Whatever you do, try to be true to your own feelings.

12

WHEN BABIES GET SICK OR

NEED HOSPITALIZATION

If your breastfed baby becomes sick and it's possible for him to swallow, you should continue nursing. He will continue to need the hydration, nourishment, and comfort that he gets from nursing while the illness runs its course or while he undergoes treatment for whatever condition he has.

Colds

Babies with nasal congestion often have a hard time nursing because of difficulty with breathing. There are several steps that you can take to relieve this congestion. These will not only make nursing easier, they will lessen the chance that your baby's mucus congestion will give rise to a bacterial infection because the mucus isn't moving out of the nose at the rate that it should.

Make sure that the air in the room where your baby spends the most time is not too dry, as dry air will aggravate his nasal congestion. You can do this by following these tips:

- Run a cool-mist vaporizer near where your baby sleeps.

- Be sure to clean your vaporizer one or two times per week. You can use a bleach solution (half a cup of bleach to a gallon of water) or whatever the manufacturer suggests.

- Take him into your bathroom after you have created a steam environment by running a hot shower with the door closed. The steam will help to drain his nasal congestion.

- Add a pinch of salt to a cup of warm tap water and, with a plastic eyedropper, squirt a few drops into each of your baby's nostrils while he is held in a sitting position (by you or someone else). Wash the eyedropper after each use. If you don't already have an eyedropper, there are saline nose sprays available at pharmacies prescription-free.

- Use a nasal aspirator or ear syringe to suction mucus from your baby's nostrils. Squeezing the rubber bulb first, insert the tip into his nostril far enough to establish a good seal, and then slowly release the bulb so that the suction will pull out loose mucus.

If you notice that your baby is just too congested to swallow enough milk to stay hydrated, you can express some milk and give it to him with a tiny cup.

Avoid medicated nasal drops and sprays, decongestants, and antihistamines. All have been shown to be potentially dangerous to babies, and none works as well as the salt solutions recommended above.

Diarrhea

A healthy breastfed baby's poop is loose, yellow, and has the consistency of pea soup. It has a slightly yeasty odor, but it doesn't stink. Diarrhea, on the other hand, is quite watery and foul-smelling. A baby with a gastrointestinal infection may have diarrhea twelve or more times within a day. Sometimes you might find a tinge of blood in the baby's diaper as well.

Whatever the degree of severity of your baby's diarrhea, continue breastfeeding, keeping close track of his weight. Weigh him undressed each morning before a feeding. If he isn't losing weight, feeds well, and is playful, he is likely to be doing fine. If he's listless and has lost five percent of his weight, call your pediatrician, as your baby is probably dehydrated and needs help.

Babies may sometimes get diarrhea as an allergic reaction to a new food that they cannot tolerate. If you suspect this, try eliminating the food to see if that solves the problem.

Another possible cause for watery poops, particularly if your baby is also acting fussy and seems to have belly cramps, is that he is getting too high a proportion of foremilk and not enough of the higher-fat-content hindmilk. This can happen if you are switching your baby to your second breast before the first is well emptied. If this is the problem, it's good to keep the baby much longer on the first breast before moving to the next.

Gastroesophageal Reflux Disease

Most babies spit up occasionally during their first weeks of life. This happens because the sphincters at the entrance to the stomach of a young baby are still young and weak, allowing just-swallowed milk (and sometimes stomach acid as well) to flow up into the esophagus. Stomach acid is very irritating to the delicate lining of the esophagus and causes the discomfort that we know as "heartburn." When this happens occasionally, it's nothing to worry about; it's part of being a baby. However, when this kind of reflux happens at virtually every feeding, the tissue of the esophagus can become so inflamed that it becomes painful for the baby to swallow. This is called gastroesophageal reflux disease (GERD), and it occurs in about three percent of babies.

GERD is very distinct from normal spitting up. Some infants with GERD vomit more than four or five times every day and spend most of their waking hours during their first weeks of life screaming in pain. Others don't vomit this much, because their stomach acid moves up into the esophagus but is never thrown up. This is known as "silent reflux." Nevertheless, the irritation is still taking place; the baby with silent reflux may have as many problems feeding as the one who vomits several times a day.

Babies with reflux disease are not able to settle at the breast, suckle until they are satisfied, or enjoy the feeling of a full tummy. They may cry as they approach the breast, take a few swallows, and start coughing and choking. They often turn their heads to the side or arch their backs while feeding, stretching their bodies out as flat as possible instead of cuddling up and melting into your body. When they throw up, they usually lose most of what they have just swallowed. Babies with GERD cry and scream during and after feedings, and they may have frequent episodes of hiccups. Some of them will also breathe with a rattling sound from the chest. Babies with a severe form of the condition may come to associate pain with feeding and thus resist it.

The scariest symptom suffered by babies with severe GERD is sleep apnea. These babies may have episodes in which they stop breathing for short periods of time while they are asleep.

Because of the symptoms that I have named, babies with GERD are sometimes mistakenly thought to have "colic." The problem with this misdiagnosis is that it may not lead to a solution of the problem.

Many babies with GERD can be helped with some fairly simple strategies:

- Avoid dressing your baby in a garment with an elastic waistband.

- Feed him in a position that puts his head well above his bottom. Experiment with pillows, if necessary, to find one that helps prop him into position.

- Try giving your baby a breastfeeding tea made up of caraway seed, fennel seed, stinging nettle, and anise seed. Give it warm (body temperature), testing the temperature on the inside of your own wrist. This can be given at any age, but I would sterilize the tea water by boiling it first for five minutes for a baby younger than six months.

- When changing a diaper, do it on a surface that is slightly raised on the "head" end, and avoid lifting the baby's legs during the process. You can roll him onto his side instead.

- Put a small wedge under the head end of the place where your baby sleeps.

- Swaddling may help calm your baby and soothe his crying.

- Give him shorter, more frequent feedings, as this may reduce the incidence of vomiting and the esophageal irritation.

- If you have plenty of milk, consider feeding him at only one breast at each feeding, paying attention to how this affects his condition.

- If your diet includes dairy products, try a dairy-free diet for two weeks. (This strategy has helped many women, but please be aware that you might not see the benefits from it until several days have passed.)

- Eliminate caffeine from your diet for two weeks.

- Eliminate wheat products from your diet for two weeks.

- Some GERD babies are helped if you give them a pacifier to suck on between feedings. Don't overdo it, but the pacifier may give you enough minutes of calm and quiet to brush your hair and to attend to your own needs or those of an older child.

If your baby's weight gain is quite slow and his condition doesn't improve with the above measures, it would be wise to see a pediatrician for an accurate diagnosis (I would recommend that you do this even before buying an over-the-counter antacid product). There are several prescription medications that may help your baby, including cimetidine (brand name: Tagamet), aluminum with magnesium hydroxide (Gaviscon), ranitidine (Zantac), aluminum hydroxide (Mylanta), omeprazole (Prilosec), and lansoprazole (Prevacid). Be aware that some of these products may have the side effect of constipation. Babies with severe GERD sometimes need to be on medication for several years.

If at all possible, continue breastfeeding; your baby with GERD will usually continue to suffer the same problems when given a cow's milk formula, without receiving the benefits of your breast milk. If your baby does wean himself, do not blame yourself for this. If you feel criticized by family members and friends who give you advice or comments, realize that they have not been in your particular situation and that they probably don't understand why what they say is hurting you.

The good news about GERD is that your baby's problem can be managed and treated. Unfortunately, there is often no quick fix. You will need as much help as you can find, because the sleep deprivation and stress associated with caring for a baby with GERD can be serious enough to put women into postpartum depression. Some mothers of GERD babies talk about how this condition delayed their developing feelings of love for the babies until the symptoms began to subside. If you have such feelings, you are not alone. I suggest that you seek out other women who have had babies with GERD; for instance, you can visit the following websites: www.reflux.org and www.cryingoverspiltmilk.co.nz.

There is life after GERD, but it may take time to get there.

Vomiting

Besides normal spitting up, you may now and then see what is called projectile vomiting—the kind when your baby vomits with such force that it sprays two or three feet away. Sometimes a baby who is overfed or squeezed around the midsection shortly after being fed will have an episode or two of projectile vomiting without there being something really wrong. Don't worry about this.

However, if projectile vomiting continues to happen and your baby begins to lose weight and his skin looks wrinkled and dry, these may be indications that he has a condition called pyloric stenosis (baby boys have it more often than girls). With this condition, there is a narrowing of the tube between the stomach and the intestines, which makes it hard for milk to move out of the stomach, so out it comes—suddenly. Pyloric stenosis most often becomes noticeable between two and eight weeks of age. A simple nonemergency surgery can correct the condition, and usually the baby can go back to breastfeeding within a few hours afterward.

If Your Baby Is Hospitalized

If your baby should ever be hospitalized, your breastfeeding relationship is going to be one of the most important elements in his healing.

Think of it this way: Your baby suddenly finds his life turned upside down. It will probably seem to him that grown-ups are no longer trustworthy! They keep coming at him with needles and sharp things, and soon enough he may start thinking that nearly every person who enters the room wants to hurt or irritate him. Breastfeeding will be the only pleasurable activity for a baby who has just had surgery or undergone some other painful medical procedure. Fortunate, then, is the baby who is breastfed, because your breast will continue to be a source of comfort and solace for him when he feels unsafe. Hopefully, the hospital staff will understand the importance of your baby's continued breastfeeding during hospitalization and will help meet your needs.

If your baby is so sick that he is unable to swallow for a time, express and store your milk. You should do this at least five times per day. This is particularly important if you are not always able to be by your baby's side at the hospital; it will help keep your milk supply up and will allow your baby to have milk ready for him when he can take it.

My own godson, Mason, was diagnosed with a cancerous tumor of the kidney. His story is particularly close to my heart because I had attended his birth and the births of both of his parents. His experiences show how important breast milk can be to hospitalized babies and also how important it is to have the help of supportive health-care professionals. His mother, Laura, tells their story:

Laura: *For me, breastfeeding wasn't a political statement or part of an alternative lifestyle, it was just the normal thing to do. I knew that breastfeeding for at least one year was the current recommendation, and I hadn't really thought much about the need to nurse beyond that—until Mason's illness was diagnosed.*

Two weeks before his first birthday, he started pushing away his food (something he had never done before). Over the next few days he pretty much stopped eating altogether, but he was still nursing. The less he ate, the more he would nurse. During this time, we asked the advice of our neighbor, a physician's assistant. She agreed with us that likely it was constipation. Over that weekend I tried all the home remedies you could name to move his bowels. Things were moving out, but still nothing was going in. He was still nursing, though, so he was hydrated and relatively well nourished.

I made an appointment Monday morning to see our pediatrician.

Upon first examination and my description of Mason's symptoms, he agreed it was some sort of bowel obstruction. A second examination, which included X rays and an ultrasound, revealed that he had a large growth in his abdomen. We went straight to a large children's hospital, where specialists diagnosed a cancerous Wilms' tumor of the kidney. It was so large (more than two pounds, and about the size of a child's football) that it was pinching the large intestine.

Mason underwent a six-hour surgery the next day. That's when I learned that, in general, breastfed infants can be nursed up to three hours prior to surgery. Formula is stopped at six hours, solid foods at eight. I was glad to be breastfeeding; it's very hard to explain to a sick one-year-old why he can't eat. After his major abdominal surgery, Mason wasn't allowed even a sip of water for forty-eight hours. When it was time to reintroduce liquids, he was insatiable; he drank every last drop we offered. After a couple of hours, once the Pedialyte stayed down, the staff said I could nurse him. They would have made him wait another twenty-four hours for formula. Once again I was glad I was nursing.

When Mason first came out of surgery, he spent the day almost comatose; he was worn out from anesthesia and the traumatic process of being in this strange place, where strange people were allowed to poke and prod him—where even his own parents helped hold him down for an IV to be set up. (There are less traumatic ways for doing this, but they take time. This was an emergency; the tumor could have leaked cancerous cells.) My son could understand little or nothing of his situation. He couldn't talk yet, couldn't tell us how he felt. When he finally started to come around, he seemed to glare at the world around him. "What is this new place, when can we leave?" he seemed to ask. Finally he was allowed to nurse. Ahh, his mother did love him. He became as needy as a newborn and wouldn't let me out of his sight.

We were told Mason might be in the hospital for two weeks, but we were discharged in six days. We were told it could take until the end of the week for him to keep down solid food, but he was eating ravenously by day three. I credit much of this rapid healing to breastfeeding. Formula and cow's milk are very heavy and hard to digest. Breast milk offered the perfect primer to get Mason's stomach going again. Once he was eating well and food was passing through without any trouble, we were free to go home.

The following week, we started both radiation and chemotherapy.

The radiation therapy lasted one week, and chemo lasted six months. There were many times when Mason would eat nothing but toast and breast milk, and he managed to maintain his weight.

There were many doctors who didn't think I should be breastfeeding him anymore. They didn't give much credit to the benefits of his nursing after the first year. This was very disheartening. I had trusted my son's life to these doctors, and they made my efforts seem insignificant or even damaging. One doctor actually thought breastfeeding was having a negative-calorie effect (that Mason was using more calories to get the milk than the milk provided him). These doctors wanted me to wean Mason and give him cow's milk or PediaSure (which is cow's milk with lots of sugar!). This proves to me that if you are having any problems or doubts about nursing, you should seek professional breastfeeding help, either through a nutritionist or lactation consultant. We were very lucky to have a professional nutritionist assigned to us. She stuck up for us with the doctors and even had my milk analyzed. (She was able to determine that it was more nutritious than cow's milk.) Mason was the only child under four I saw in the oncology clinic who didn't have a nasogastric tube (a feeding tube that goes through the nose to the stomach, used for bypassing the mouth in people who can't or won't eat). Mason was able to gain just enough weight not to need one. I can't help but wonder how big a part breastfeeding played.

If your baby needs to be hospitalized, it's important that those who will be caring for him are familiar with the importance of breastfeeding for your baby (and you) and will see to your needs. Best are the hospitals that provide sleeping facilities so you don't have to sit in a hard chair all night to be near your baby. Keep up your commitment to breastfeeding, and arrange for all the support you can get. Returning to breastfeeding will help your baby recover his health more quickly. If your pediatrician tries to convince you to stop nursing your sick baby, you might want to seek a nutritionist's support like Laura did.

13

WEANING

There is no "best" age to wean a baby. Women in different cultures wean their babies at different times, usually according to what is best for the babies in view of the local food supply. In many countries where poverty is rampant and food is scarce, children are nursed by their mothers and grandmothers until they are three or four or even older. A long nursing period helps make an easier, healthier transition between the diet available to the toddler and that eaten by adults. There is no reason, however, why a mother living in a country where food is plentiful must automatically wait to wean until her toddler refuses the breast. At the same time, if your baby is gaining and developing well, and both you and your baby are still enjoying nursing, there is no good reason why you should stop.

Do I sound like a moderate on this issue? I hope so, because I do think there is a middle course between obligatory weaning by a certain age, which is chosen by someone besides you and your baby, and nursing for as long as your toddler wants, even when she is inflicting real damage on your body. What do I mean by damage? I'm talking about cracked, bleeding nipples caused not by a young baby who hasn't got the latch right yet but by someone with teeth who could be chewing food instead of chewing on you. I'm talking about bruises to your arms and legs caused by your toddler kicking you in anger because you didn't teach her nursing manners at a younger age.

At the risk of being accused of promoting parental cruelty, I do want to point out that all mammals eventually wean their young. In some species, the weaning process has much to do with the size of the baby. A young elephant, for instance, will reach a size when it would have to get on its knees to gain access to mother's milk. Once young pigs get fat enough (and it's not unusual for a sow to give birth to twelve in a litter), the litter is no longer able to fit into nursing position at once. In addition, once the adult teeth start appearing, most mammalian mothers no longer find joy in continuing to nurture their whopping offspring, so mother-led weaning is the norm. Please understand, though, that I am an advocate of continuing to nurse your human baby through teething and beyond—as long as it is the best for both of you.

One of my midwife friends nursed her three children until they were each six or seven years old. Her decision to nurse this long did not stem from a parenting philosophy that everyone should do this but rather from the fact that her husband suffered from a variety of very serious allergies. She worried that their children might inherit this tendency from him and so decided that they would benefit from as long a nursing period as possible. All were gentle nursers, she told me, so she never had to deal with biting or other problems having to do with nursing an older child. When her oldest child, a daughter, was six years old, my friend began asking her if she didn't think she was old enough now to think of weaning. "But, Mom," her daughter said, "you're always talking on the phone to women about how good breast milk is. Don't you think it's good for me too?" Certainly in this case, and I'm sure in many others, child-led weaning was the best strategy for the family. Not long after this conversation, my friend's daughter decided that she was ready to give up nursing.

Some children can be quite tenacious—and creative—in clinging to nursing when their mother is ready to wean. I know of a case in which the mother had made several attempts to wean her robust two-and-a-half-year-old boy, without success. Finally, her husband convinced her that if she went away with her girlfriends for a weekend, the transition could be made. The night after she left, he was surprised to find that his enterprising little son had joined the litter of puppies nursing on their mother on the front porch. I laughed so hard hearing that one that I forgot to ask when and how the dog weaned him.

Another tenacious lad was the one that Mary Breckinridge, founder of the famous Frontier Nursing Service, described in her fascinating autobiography, *Wide Neighborhoods.* When asked about the health of the Appalachian babies the Frontier Nursing Service midwives delivered, she said, "We will find it hard to cope with our babies if they become any more mentally and physically abusive than many of them are now. Not so long ago, a woman with an eighteen-month-old boy came to our hospital outpatient clinic at Hyden Hospital and sat down to nurse him. The Medical Director said to her, 'Don't you think it is time to wean your baby?'

" 'Yes, I know, Doc,' she replied, 'I know, but every time I try to, he throws rocks at me.' "

One of my favorite weaning stories comes from a midwife who remembers her grandmother, who lived on a midwestern farm in the 1940s. The women of the family were exchanging weaning stories, and the grandmother began telling how she weaned her youngest son after he was old enough to be rough with her. Anticipating that he would want a drink soon, she went over to the woodstove, covered her hand with the soot that had accumulated inside the stove lid, unbuttoned her dress, and rubbed the soot on her breasts. Her son toddled in and she opened her dress top. Horrified at the sight of her blackened breasts, he cried, "What happened?"

"Pigs got 'em," she replied. He never wanted to nurse again.

Partial weaning begins as soon as your baby starts eating some solid foods along with nursing, usually by the age of six to eight months. Sometimes a baby about the age of ten or eleven months will wean herself completely after she has been partially weaned for a few weeks. There is no reason to fight this tendency by insisting that a baby this old continue to nurse if she clearly doesn't want to. On the other hand, her refusal to nurse may be temporary. If she starts to nurse again in earnest, she is likely to restimulate your milk supply. In addition, your baby may want to nurse more than usual if you are traveling with her, even if she has started to wean herself.

If your baby does seem to be weaning herself, you have the choice of whether to wean her to the bottle or the cup. One disadvantage of weaning to the bottle is that there will have to be a second weaning, from the bottle to the cup. Another is that a child who depends upon taking a bottle to bed every time she takes a nap or before she goes to bed each night is more likely to develop cavities than the child who gets her drinking done in a faster manner. The slow drip of sweet liquid, including milk, promotes tooth decay.

You can wean your baby to a cup as early as the age of seven or eight months. Since cups can spill unnoticed, you will have to pay special attention to getting enough liquid into her. This means that you will have to sit down with her and help her to control the flow of liquid from the cup so she doesn't pour her milk or juice onto the floor or up her nose. If you notice that your baby seems to get dehydrated (some symptoms are a depressed fontanel and dry-looking skin), you need to get her to take more liquid. Increase the amount she gets by either sitting patiently with her and giving her drinks from a cup or by switching her to a bottle.

It is preferable for weaning to take place when both you and your baby are feeling healthy and well rested. In the best-case scenario, it can happen so gradually that you and your baby are not at all upset by it. You may find it easiest to eliminate one feeding at a time over a several-week period. Find something interesting to do with your baby at the time of the feeding that you want to eliminate. This could range from giving her a drink from a cup to taking a walk. The idea is to break the usual routine with an interesting new activity that will distract your baby from the fact that she's not nursing.

If you usually nurse your baby to sleep, try this instead: Give her a big hug and kiss, lie her gently down in her bed, and pat her back for a while. She is used to having long periods of physical closeness and cuddling as she nurses, so it's good to give her plenty of physical attention during the weaning process. She needs to know that she will still get loving attention from you when she's not nursing.

By the time you are down to one feeding a day and you're finished with night feedings, most of the weaning process has already happened. Some babies might cling to that last feeding for a few weeks or even months after having eliminated the rest, while many others seem ready and able to wean completely.

Some mothers find that it's quite easy for them to eliminate daytime feedings and not so easy when it comes to the nighttime feedings. It helps if you get your baby's father to answer your baby's cries for a nighttime feed. He can cuddle your baby and explain that Mom's asleep now and it's time to go back to bed. If he thinks the baby might be thirsty, he can offer a sip of water. It's important to realize that this strategy will work only if you and your partner are convinced that you are not being cruel parents by refusing to continue nighttime feedings.

I remember one couple who both felt it was time to wean their two-year-old daughter. For four months, this toddler had wanted to nurse only at night. At first, her mother didn't resent these nightly wake-ups, because the toddler was sweet about nursing and always went right back to sleep. By four months later, the girl began demanding to sleep in her parents' bed. She was a finicky sleeper in the family bed, and she would wake up and scream if her mother so much as turned over. This situation needed to change, and the couple decided that their daughter should return to sleeping in her own room. And, since it was unlikely that she would wean herself if her mother kept responding to her—since her mother only reminded her of how much she wanted to nurse—the husband decided that he should be the one to respond to her nightly wake-ups. The next night, when the toddler woke up crying in her bedroom, he was the one who went to her. The first night she cried and carried on, and the second night he even had to pace the floor with her for a while so that she would calm down. By the third night, she barely whimpered, and after that, she began sleeping through the night.

Single mothers have more difficulty with weaning because it's more difficult for them to obtain this kind of help. If you're single, you may need to enlist the help of a dear friend whom your baby already knows to spend the night at your place and respond to baby's nighttime food requests.

The main thing to remember about weaning is that your baby's attitude toward weaning will be greatly affected by your own. If you are not emotionally ready for weaning, there's a very good chance that your baby will not be ready either. If you think that weaning is going to mean a terrible loss for your baby, you might as well nurse for as long as it takes for you to be able to make a smooth transition.

14

SHARED NURSING, WET-NURSING,
AND FORGOTTEN LORE

When breastfeeding becomes marginalized in a culture, maternal behavior that was considered normal in times when people grew up seeing breastfeeding women around them comes to be viewed as socially unacceptable. Shared nursing and wet-nursing are examples of behaviors that have been common all over the world in nonurbanized societies. Unfortunately, when bottle-feeding of artificial milks becomes the primary mode of infant feeding, how people used to relate to one another can rather quickly be forgotten, and many begin to think that breastfeeding is—and should remain—an essentially private experience between each mother and her baby. Not only that, the marginalization of breastfeeding means that knowledge about the very capacities of women's bodies to lactate gets lost to a surprising extent to women themselves and to medical professionals. In this chapter, I'll explore these themes, their relevance to our own times, and the way I was able to regain some of the forgotten knowledge that it is still useful to have.

Shared Nursing

The first summer we settled on our land in Tennessee, we were presented with our first nursing challenge: One hundred of the three hundred of us came down with hepatitis A—probably from eating uncooked watercress that had been put in the store. Two pregnant women, Linda and Lisa, had their babies prematurely because of contracting the disease. Both babies were too small to maintain their body temperature, even in the August heat, so each spent some weeks in incubators at our local hospital. Hospital policy in the nursery at that time didn't allow for mothers to even hold their babies, let alone nurse them, so both were given formula milk by bottle for the duration of their hospital stay. It was clear to me that the main way we could help Linda and Lisa was to keep their milk flowing so that when their babies were finally discharged, they would be able to switch from formula given by bottle to drinking their mothers' milk directly from the breast. I hadn't yet heard of "nipple confusion," so I didn't know that babies sometimes become lazy about nursing because of habits they form from bottle-feeding, and I didn't foresee any problems. Breast-pump technology was in its infancy in the early 1970s; we had some manual pumps of the old bicycle-horn type, but nothing like the electric pumps of today. I did know that milk had to be regularly removed from each mother's breasts to keep up milk production. Although Linda and Lisa had some degree of success pumping manually, it was obvious that stronger measures would be necessary for them to maintain good milk production. At my suggestion, some of the other mothers of young babies in our community worked out schedules among themselves and helped Linda and Lisa keep their milk supply abundant by bringing their own babies to their homes to be nursed by them.

Perhaps because in 1971 the very act of breastfeeding a baby was considered a radical thing to do, it didn't seem to us much more radical to occasionally nurse one another's babies if and when it became necessary. This arrangement certainly helped Linda and Lisa keep their milk flowing, emptying their breasts far better than they could achieve with the manual pumps. After discharge from the hospital, Linda's baby, who had been the smaller of the two, required some supplementation with formula for a while, but both of the preemies were eventually able to breastfeed exclusively.

When women have strong friendships, trust one another, are healthy, and live close together, breastfeeding one another's children occasionally can be convenient and helpful. In the early years of our community, the overall budget didn't permit us to build single-family dwellings, so our solution was to build some houses that were large enough to be shared by three or four families and some single people as well. Under these circumstances, close friendships developed among many of the women. We midwives, for instance, all had young babies during the early years; when we were called out to a birth, we couldn't always take our babies with us, so one of our housemates would ordinarily make sure they were fed. If my baby was asleep and not yet ready for a feeding when I was on a lecture tour in our large bus (accompanied by a rock band and their families), I would feed the baby who was awake and most ready to eat, and that baby's mother would then feed my baby when he woke up. As one of my friends put it, "It seemed like a pretty natural part of life, especially among us women who knew each other so well and were so comfortable with each other. It was occasional for most but just not a big deal."

At the same time, the women of my community did find it necessary to develop an etiquette surrounding shared nursing. We agreed, for instance, that asking to breastfeed another woman's baby out of mere curiosity was impolite and intrusive and shouldn't be done.

On the other hand, I remember how much I ached to have a live baby at my breast during the first days of grief I experienced after the death of my prematurely born son in 1971. I don't remember now if the mother of one of the babies whose birth I had most recently assisted offered that I could nurse her baby or if I dared to ask her permission, but I do know that I nursed her daughter for a few healing minutes when I was still raw with grief. My son's death had made me understand in a visceral way why grieving mothers sometimes steal someone else's baby; those few moments soothed something very deep in me, and my healing began.

A few years later we had a situation in my community that called for helpful intervention. A woman named Eileen had given birth to surprise twin girls ten weeks early. Each baby weighed 3 pounds 5 oz. (1,500 g). One of the girls had respiratory-distress syndrome followed by pneumonia and needed to be on a respirator for almost a week. Eileen pumped her milk nine times a day and brought it to the nursery where the girls were being kept. First the babies were tube-fed, and then, when they got stronger, they were bottle-fed. Both babies were well under five pounds when they came home and were mainly bottle-fed Eileen's milk (with only one nursing per day). Eileen eventually quit pumping and began nursing them a lot, and they quickly began to prefer nursing.

The twins did well, but Eileen and her husband, Matthew, were bleary-eyed with exhaustion. Around this time there was another crisis, involving a first-time single mother, Karen, whose baby died because of a prolapsed cord at the onset of labor (Karen's lower limbs had been paralyzed by polio during childhood). It occurred to me that the two women might be able to help each other, if they lived in the same house and all were open to the idea of Karen helping to nurse the twins. The three adults agreed to try this.

Karen: *I moved to Eileen and Matthew's house and was handed a hungry baby right away. I remember it being awkward at first, because I didn't really know these people nor did I know how to nurse a baby. I learned fast. The girls were always ready to eat. By the time I got to them, they were two months old and around six pounds each. At first my nipples got very sore, so I used a nipple shield. But the twins didn't like it, and I soon got used to them nursing. The twins would nurse for hours, regardless of my milk supply. I could nurse them both while lying on my back, propping them up with pillows. I loved nursing; it felt good and it helped me get over the loss of my own child.*

Eileen: *It became apparent that the only way for us to do it together was as a full partnership. We both shared both twins. At night, one baby would sleep in each of our rooms, alternating which baby each night.*

Karen: *The twins grew fast. Their bony butts filled out, and they were actually fat by five months old. My love for the family grew too. They let me help care for their babies, which is what I most needed at that time in my life, and I gave them the help they needed. Eileen and I naturally had different parenting styles, but we respected each other and helped balance one another out—keeping each other clear of all the pitfalls of a first mothering experience.*

The twins did not seem to care that one of their mothers was

biological and one was not. When they started to talk, we were both "Momma." People remarked on how much the twins looked like me, which is understandable, since they spent many hours staring at my face. The twins are grown women now. I am grateful that such an intimate and compassionate arrangement could happen and that everyone could be the better for it.

Sometimes nursing someone else's baby is a one-time-only event. I can remember a birth to a single mother after a long, exhausting labor. After an hour or so spent trying to get her baby to latch, she was becoming frustrated, which was preventing her baby from calming down enough to take her breast. Noticing that she was near tears, I finally asked if she'd mind if I showed her baby by letting him latch on to my breast. (It was the quickest thing I could think of, as I hadn't yet been able to talk her through steps that would work for her.)

"Would you, please?" she asked. After a few sucks at my breast—and a perfect latch—her newborn son was handed back to her. He, now calm and having learned what to do, latched on to her breast without hesitation.

Problem-solving during the early days sometimes went like this, especially when mother and baby were having trouble getting the hang of nursing and both were getting frustrated. The women in my community were generally aware that:

- When a new mother has trouble getting her new baby to latch correctly, an experienced baby can efficiently teach her what a correct latch should feel like.

- When a new baby is having a difficult time latching correctly and there is no lactation consultant available, time and frustration can be saved by having an experienced, healthy mother teach her.

I'm sure that we avoided many cases of sore nipples in this way during the early days, when we hadn't yet learned about other techniques for dealing with this type of problem.

The following story illustrates how a sisterly relationship made one baby's hard transition into life a little sweeter.

Malika: *After my sister-in-law had a traumatic delivery in the hospital, the nurses insisted that the baby be given formula due to low blood sugar. My phone rang at 3:00 A.M., with my sister-in-law's pleading voice on the line. Her pediatrician had reluctantly agreed to let her baby have my breast milk instead of formula. So, with my infant son in one arm and breast milk in the other, we trekked into the nursery in the wee hours of the morning. The nurse blankly stared at me in disbelief when I announced that I was there with milk for my nephew. She had such a prissy look on her face that I offered to nurse him instead. "Oh, that won't be necessary," she said, and took it from me with gloved hands, all the while repeatedly telling me this was against policy and that she was very unsure of it. I watched her feed my nephew, who clearly loved it and was very grateful. The worried look disappeared from his face. The good thing was that he didn't need formula after all, because his mom was able to nurse him not long after he got my milk.*

Malika's story also illustrates how widely attitudes vary about mother's milk in our country—not so much regionally but rather among individuals. To some (including me), breast milk is the perfect food for babies and, as such, it is different from every other secretion of the body; nothing else we secrete is food. Others worry about it precisely *because* it comes from the body, and they are not differentiating between food and other bodily fluids.

I had thought until recently that the women of The Farm were perhaps the only women in the United States who sometimes shared milk with one another's babies. After all, the websites for the Centers for Disease Control and La Leche League both discourage the practice, citing the possibility that another mother might have a serious contagious disease. It is certainly understandable why the CDC and LLL have not given their stamp of approval to informal arrangements for the sharing of human milk, given that breastfeeding is considered a possible way of transmitting the HIV (AIDS) virus. Both the CDC and LLL recommend that any mother needing human milk for her baby, who can't provide her own, should buy it as a prescription item through a human milk bank. However, given the high price of human milk obtained at such banks in the United States (three dollars per ounce) and the average three-month-old baby's need for twenty-five to thirty ounces per day, the cost is clearly prohibitive for many mothers who nevertheless want the benefits of breast milk for their babies. Shared-nursing arrangements are particularly useful to adoptive mothers who haven't been able to successfully induce lactation and to mothers whose previous breast surgery interferes with milk production or transfer. Women in these situations may make arrangements with trusted friends or relatives who can provide breast milk, saving themselves the steep costs of milk banks.

I have noticed, however, that in recent years a growing number of breastfeeding mothers have been telling stories of sharing their milk with one another's babies in different publications and on the Internet.[1-3] Such arrangements are usually made on an informal basis involving family members, close friends, or neighbors who are in a position to know one another's health status. There are several factors behind this trend. First, it shows that many women have accepted the message that breast milk is the best food for babies. Second, the Internet offers many ways for women to share information, stories, and ideas. Third, the short unpaid maternity leave for most U.S. women (with a general lack of employer accommodation for breastfeeding) has motivated some mothers to seek a way to make sure their babies receive breast milk.

In some families, the practice of women sharing nursing is part of a culture that has been long accepted. Brenda explains:

Brenda: *I am the youngest of five children—four girls and one boy. All of my siblings, including my brother's wife, had natural births and breastfed. We all helped each other out with child care. Our children were often close in age and breastfeeding at the same time. If we were watching our sister's or sister-in-law's baby and it was hungry, we breastfed it. This was just common sense. The baby was satisfied, and the mom didn't need to worry while she was away. These children played together, grew up together, and still maintain close relationships. They have a great deal of fun together now as adults.*

Another relationship was that of a thirty-year-old Tucson mother who offered this service to her sister, whose prematurely born baby needed breast milk just as much as his mother needed the income from her job as a waitress. Since her employer wasn't willing to make arrangements that would allow her to continue nursing her baby during the day, this woman's sister nursed the baby (as needed) while she was at work. In quick trips to the bathroom, the mother was able to manually express enough milk at work to relieve her overfull breasts, and she nursed her baby at night. The cooperation between the two women eased a difficult situation for the working sister and her baby.

Muslim societies recognize the special closeness of babies who have been nourished at the same breasts, even when the babies are not related

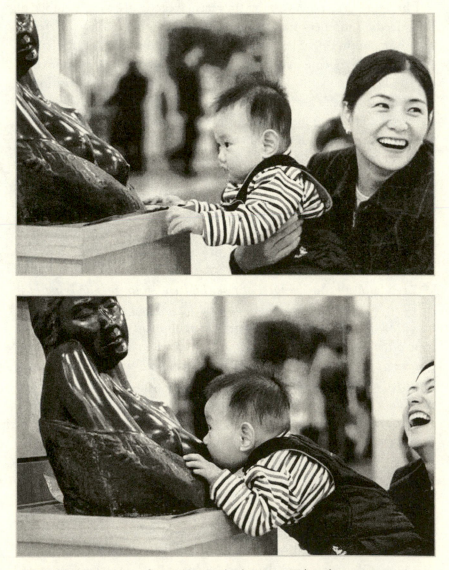

Breastfed babies are often curious and adventurous when they see attractive breasts.

by blood. From the Muslim perspective, because milk is so close to blood, the relationship of babies who share the same mother's milk is considered to be as close as that between siblings. This means that a young woman who would have to be veiled in the presence of any men outside of her immediate family would not be required to wear the veil in the presence of a "milk sibling." Milk siblings should not marry each other, for this same reason.

Shared nursing may not appeal to every mother, nor is it practical for many women. At the same time, in some situations and cultures, shared nursing involving women with no communicable diseases makes sense and promotes a tender closeness between the women who share this aspect of their mothering. HIV testing would seem to me a sensible precaution before embarking upon such an arrangement.

Wet-Nursing

We know from written and pictorial records that for centuries women in various parts of the world have nursed babies besides their own. Wet-nursing was a common feature of life in ancient civilizations such as Babylon, Mesopotamia, Egypt, and Sumeria, according to several references dating from the third millennium B.C. These range from ancient lullabies to legal contracts between families and wet nurses. A contract might, for instance, spell out the length of time that the hired wet nurse would be expected to nurse the child and might specify that she was not to become pregnant or suckle another child (including her own) during that period. If midwifery was women's first profession, wet-nursing was probably the second.

Who were these wet nurses, and how were they able to do their jobs? We know that in any given population some women can produce so much milk that they can feed several babies with ease. According to Jane Sharp, seventeenth-century English midwife and author, "Some women...are so well tempered to increase milk that they can suckle a child of their own, and another for a friend; and it will not hurt their own child." Presumably, many women with this ability must have found employment as wet nurses. In sixteenth- and seventeenth-century England, nearly all of the wet nurses were married women living with their husbands, with children of their own. Some may have had to abandon their own babies to another's care while they served as wet nurse for the baby of someone who could pay them. Some of the earlier references tell of wet-nursing without any commercial relationship between the two women. The Old Testament story of Ruth, for instance, tells of Ruth giving her son to her mother-in-law, Naomi, to nurse.

Not surprisingly, the practice of using wet nurses (whether or not they were paid for their services) seems to have been especially common among royalty and people of wealth. Women who were poor or penniless probably had little choice about taking up wet-nursing in many cases. One of the reasons why some royal families employed wet nurses during times past was that people knew a woman's return to fertility could be delayed by exclusively nursing her baby. Giving a newborn to a wet nurse would hasten the queen's next conception and make it possible for her to give birth to more royal heirs than would have been likely had she nursed all of her children herself.

It might surprise some people to know that wet-nursing is not a thing of the long-ago past in many parts of the world. I learned this in 1965 while working for a few weeks in a Chinese boatbuilder's yard in Penang, Malaysia. The boatbuilder's wife had given birth to a baby a few months previously. I remember her situation as being somewhat unusual (for me), since her baby was being wet-nursed elsewhere in Penang and wouldn't rejoin his biological family until he was weaned during his second year of life. This middle-class family took the wet-nursing option because they believed that human milk was far superior to artificial formula milk, which was being heavily promoted to Malaysian families at the time, but they also believed that it would require too much of the mother's energy to nurse her own baby.

Wet-nursing is making a modest comeback in the United States, for the same reasons that shared-nursing arrangements are being made. A Los Angeles–based agency serves women who can afford to hire a wet nurse, typically at a rate of $1,000 per week. One such wet nurse nursed ten babies over the previous seven years as a way of funding her own children's college educations. Asked if she thought less of herself for earning money in this way, she answered that she found it fulfilling.[4]

As China has modernized, breastfeeding and wet-nursing rates have dropped rapidly—more women have returned to work soon after giving birth, and infant-formula companies' aggressive marketing techniques have reached more people. However, the poisoned-infant-milk scandal that erupted in September 2008 sparked a reconsideration of the worth of breastfeeding and wet-nursing in China. Millions of parents found out that the infant formula they had been told was healthier than mother's milk was actually heavily contaminated with melamine, an industrial chemical meant to fool tests for protein in watered-down milk. As a result, at least six babies died from kidney stones and some 300,000 others suffered serious urinary and kidney problems that may be with them for their entire lives. Suddenly, Chinese parents, feeling betrayed by their government's food-safety agencies and many domestic infant-formula companies, began to search for women to serve as wet nurses to their babies, and lactating women began to realize that their milk was valuable enough to be advertised via the Internet. Wet-nursing clearly is making a comeback.

Forgotten Knowledge

When humans set aside a biological activity and rarely perform it in significant numbers, the knowledge of the activity within that culture can quickly vanish to a degree that is astonishing. The following story, told to me by a Dutch midwife, serves as an example of what I mean. The Netherlands, like other Western countries after World War II, moved toward widespread acceptance of bottle-feeding babies with various formulas based upon cow's milk, even though a larger proportion of the Dutch population stayed with breastfeeding than that of the United States around the same time.

The Dutch midwife told me of a conversation she had with a young woman who had recently become pregnant with her first baby. Like many Dutch women, she came to the midwife intending to have her baby at home. Typically, this would be an unmedicated birth. "That's wonderful that you are pregnant," the midwife told her. "Are you planning to breastfeed your baby?"

"Oh, no," said the young mother-to-be. "I really can't stand any pain."

"Why do you think that breastfeeding a baby is painful?" asked the midwife, surprised that someone choosing to have an unmedicated birth would be hesitant to breastfeed because of fear of pain.

"Well," replied the young woman, "don't you have to make holes in the nipple with a needle?"

Dumbfounded at first, the midwife realized—after continuing this discussion for a while longer—that when the young woman was a child she had seen her mother enlarging the hole in a rubber nipple. Having inspected her own nipples without finding any visible holes, she assumed that such holes would need to be created with a needle.

I can promise you that if this story was told anywhere in the world before 1900, it would have been hard for anyone to believe that a young adult could be so ignorant. If you told that story today to someone who grew up in a village in which every baby is breastfed, they would be amazed that someone in this day and age could know so little about her own body. And yet I have a story that illustrates that even the most highly educated authorities in our culture may have similarly breathtaking gaps in their knowledge and understanding about breasts and breastfeeding.

Five of my friends and fellow community members took an anatomy and physiology course at a college while studying to be registered nurses. While lecturing on the structure of the female breast, the instructor of the course (who had a PhD in his field) mentioned in passing that milk came out of a hole in the nipple.

"Do you really mean only one hole?" one of my friends, who had breastfed five children, asked, half-suspecting that she had heard him wrong.

"Yes," he said confidently.

One of the other women from The Farm raised her hand and tried a different approach. "But our textbook states that there are several holes in the female nipple," she said, pointing to the book on her desk.

"Oh, that's not the text that I use for my final authority," he replied. "Come down to my office after class, and I'll show you."

Worried that they would embarrass their professor before the entire class more than he had already embarrassed himself, they left the subject until the class was over, wondering all the while if he really thought that the textbook he had chosen for their course was wrong in such an important detail. Once they were all in his office, he reached for the "more authoritative" textbook from his shelves. Opening it to the crucial page, he quickly realized that he had been wrong. Finally humbled, he turned to my friends and asked, "How did you know?"

"Among us, we have breastfed seventeen children," one of the women answered for all.

This story illustrates several facts. The first may surprise many academics—not just the professor mentioned; *Women who have breast-fed are themselves an important source of knowledge about breastfeeding.* None of my friends found it necessary to read a textbook about how many holes there are in the human nipple, any more than a man would need to be told how many holes there are in his penis. They learned from observation, just as the man does. But there is a difference: Unless the woman's breast is producing colostrum or milk, she is not able to see how many holes there are in her nipples. Second—and this is a really important point—written knowledge can easily be forgotten when it is not backed up by bodily experience. No one who has ever seen milk spray from a breast could be fooled into thinking that there is only one hole in a woman's nipple.

The anatomy professor is just one example illustrating the confusion of societies in which most people live in a way that has become quite disconnected from nature.

A person who grew up on a farm would never have made this kind of mistake. Even if they had never seen a human female nursing a baby, they would have witnessed all of the farm's animals feeding their young in the way that nature intended. However, with fewer and fewer people having grown up on a family farm, ignorance of the capacities of the human body becomes more pronounced and widespread. It doesn't take very long before human abilities that were common knowledge for thousands of generations become shrouded in mystery.

Sometimes the level of ignorance is beyond what I would have thought possible. It wasn't long ago that I met a young woman, now a medical student, who had an interesting story to tell me.

Gretchen: *When I was pregnant with my first child, my nurse–midwife asked a typical prenatal question: "Are you planning on breast- or bottle-feeding?" Puzzled, I looked to my husband for guidance, as this was his third child and I relied on his experience quite a bit during the pregnancy. He emphatically suggested I at least try to breast-feed. The problem was that I didn't know what breastfeeding was. My midwife suggested I attend a La Leche League meeting during my pregnancy, as the leaders there would be able to answer any questions I had. A few days later I found myself sitting in a library meeting room surrounded by women who were feeding their babies, but not with*

bottles—the way I thought babies were fed. They were all breastfeeding. Until this point in my life, I had no idea that breasts were for feeding babies. I didn't even know we were capable of feeding babies with our breasts. This was something I don't ever recall being told, nor do I have any memory of ever seeing a woman breastfeeding a baby prior to my first La Leche League meeting. I was twenty years old and had just discovered the real purpose for breasts!

I educated myself more about breastfeeding and decided I would at least give it a try. I gave myself a goal of one year and no more. I then went on to nurse my firstborn for two and a half years, including through a pregnancy. He weaned when his sister was nine months old, and she weaned when she was about two and a half as well. I never could have imagined how important breastfeeding would be for me, and I am very thankful I have a husband who helped me discover what my breasts are really for.

In case you think I have already exhausted the modern-day fund of ignorance that plagues many highly urbanized societies, read on. Take the little-known fact that there is plenty of evidence that many women who haven't been pregnant recently can fully lactate, stimulated primarily by a baby's sucking at the breast. One of the neatest talents breasts have is that they don't really retire, or, if they do, they can be called back into service. That's right: Many grandmothers can suckle their grandchildren, if need be, and within a few days' time (usually) be able to keep up with a baby's nutritional needs. This has been the case throughout time, and there are still many groups of people who continue to hold this important cultural knowledge and use it daily to make life easier for mothers and babies.

I didn't learn about this ability from books—although it has been briefly mentioned in several texts on lactation. Generally, it is discussed with reference to women in nonliterate societies or from the distant past. Breastfeeding self-help books mention "induced lactation" in the context of providing strategies for women whose babies are adopted, generally advising that the mother use a lactation aid, a variety of medications, and breast pumps. Even so, most people in our culture would be amazed to find out that it is possible for some women to produce milk even if they have not recently (or ever) been pregnant and given birth.

My own first experience with a baby being nursed by someone other than her mother took place in Malaysia during the 1960s when I was in the Peace Corps. Shortly after our arrival in Malaysia, a group of fellow volunteers and I were invited to have coffee and conversation at the home of the headman of a Malay rural village. Excited by the chance to be in a real Malay home on stilts, we climbed the ladder to the doorway one by one and were greeted by the headman and his young wife. They invited us to sit on the grass mats surrounding the low table set with coffee cups. Two older children played quietly in a corner, under the watchful eye of their grandmother. But that wasn't all that this color-fully clad woman was doing. To my complete surprise, I noticed that she was cradling and *nursing* the youngest child of the family. The Peace Corps had spent a lot of time during our training period trying to pre-pare us to live in this non-Western Muslim culture. We learned never to point with our index finger, beckon someone with our palm upward, eat with our left hand, show the soles of our feet, or pass before someone else without first crouching enough that our head would be lower than theirs. But no one had prepared me to see an elderly-looking grand-mother nursing a baby. Because her breasts were so empty-looking, I assumed that her grandchild was enjoying suckling but wasn't getting anything to drink in the process. Little did I know at that time that breasts don't have to look full to be able to deliver plenty of milk.

Years later, after I had been a midwife for ten years or so and all of my children had been nourished at my breast, I had another chance to be among women and babies from an entirely different culture. This time I was spending a couple of weeks in Lesotho, an impoverished country whose only neighbor is the Republic of South Africa. While there, it was impossible to forget that Lesotho depends heavily upon foreign aid to feed its people because of the deforestation and subsequent loss of topsoil that occurred during the colonial period a century and more ear-lier. At any rate, during my time there, I came into contact with several grandmothers who were nursing children who appeared to be three or four years old. Again, I assumed that they were not actually nourishing these children.

It wasn't until I ran across a fascinating passage in a nineteenth-century medical text a few years later that I realized I was unaware of all the capacities of women's bodies. The passage was written by M. Audebert, a well-known French obstetrician, and referred to a case he learned about in 1841:

Angeline Chaufaille, sixty-two years of age, and who had not had children for twenty-seven years, undertook to nurse her granddaughter artificially. From time to time, in order to amuse it, she presented it with her nipple, but what was her surprise when she suddenly found both her breasts full of an apparently good, healthy, and nutritive milk! She continued to nurse it for a year, and the secretion had not entirely ceased after the child had been weaned two months. At this juncture, her daughter again became a mother, her milk dried up, and the grandmother was able to nurse the second child.

When I read that passage, I realized that there was a good chance that the Malay grandmother and those older women I had seen in Lesotho had been lactating as well. What's more, none of these women had needed to use a device to deliver a substitute milk through a tube taped to their nipple in order to keep the baby stimulating the breast.

From that time on, I kept my eyes and ears open for more information on the subject. Here's what I found. Gabrielle Palmer's book, *The Politics of Breastfeeding*, references nineteenth-century England's famous Judith Waterford, whose amazing ability as a wet nurse was documented in both medical and lay publications. At the age of eighty-one, Waterford demonstrated how she could still squeeze milk from her left breast that was "nice, sweet and not different from that of young and healthy mothers." After her marriage at twenty-two, she spent the next fifty years nursing babies—six of her own, eight nurslings, and many more for friends and neighbors. By the age of seventy-five, she regretted that she could feed only one baby at a time.[5]

I also found an extensive article published in 1940 in the *Bulletin of the History of Medicine.* Its author, H. A. Wieschhoff, discovered many reports published between 1640 and 1935 of women in primitive societies in Africa, Indonesia, India, North America, South America, and New Zealand, which were familiar with, and even dependent upon, the ability of a woman to resume lactating many years past the birth of her youngest child. An English writer, for instance, who had spent time among the Lepcha people of northern India wrote: "...any woman who once has given birth to a child is believed to be able to 'produce milk spontaneously when a baby sucks.'" Among these same people, he went on, "it is the obligation of the grandmother to suckle the child should its own mother die."[6]

A German ethnologist who lived among the Xhosa people in southern Africa for more than four decades in the last half of the nineteenth century wrote that this phenomenon was common among these peoples and stated that he had learned of "numerous" cases in which women from sixty to eighty years of age were able to suckle their daughters' children or even their own great-grandchildren.

The oldest reference in the 1940 article was to a report made by a Jesuit who visited the Iroquois people in 1640 and wrote: "Here is an occurrence which many have considered remarkable. There was a woman who had had nine children, the last of whom was married, and had children; I mean to say, in a word, that this woman was very old—I believe that her age was more than 60 years; yet one of her daughters happening to die, and leaving a child in arms, this good old woman took the child and offered it her withered breast. The child, by pulling at it, caused the milk to return, so that the grandmother nourished it for more than a year."

Wieschhoff's 1940 article also mentions that Dr. David Livingstone, the medical missionary who searched for the origin of the Nile, wrote in 1858 that he had witnessed many cases during his travels in which a grandmother was able to nourish a grandchild at her breast, stating that sometimes mother and grandmother shared in suckling a baby.

The ability of elderly women in medieval Europe to lactate has also been noted in some sources. In Bologna, an elderly couple adopted an abandoned baby and, after some prayers, the wife found her breasts full of milk and was able to nurse the baby. And in Tuscany, church frescoes show the "miracle" of a seventy-five-year-old woman who was able to nurse her grandchild for several months after both parents had perished in the plague.[7]

Recently I met a young nursing student named Albert. When I asked members of his class if any of them were aware of the ability of grandmothers to lactate, he told me his story.

Albert: *My mother had a complication with my birth, so she was hospitalized for a couple of weeks. During this period, it was my grandmother who took over nursing me. She said that at the age of forty-eight,* *she would wake up in the middle of the night to feed me or change my diaper. Maybe this is the reason for the strong bond I have with my grandmother. I am actually her favorite among her grandchildren. When my mother recovered from her illness, it took some time before I was able to make the transition back to her (I know there is no rationale for this, but it just happened). They said that I would cry and cry for my grandmother.*

In case you wonder how—apparently independently of one an-other—indigenous and ancient peoples in so many parts of the world discovered that grandmothers can often lactate long past their own childbearing years, I'd like to suggest how this might be known. Many women have told me—and I have experienced this myself—that when they hear a baby cry, they sometimes feel a tingling sensation in their breasts that is very much like the feeling of milk letting down when one is already lactating. I would call this a prolactin rush. Although I have never breastfed a baby since I weaned my youngest child, I have always had the feeling that my milk would return if I tried breastfeeding. I am reasonably certain that I am not the first nor will I be the last woman to have this feeling.

Sharon, although not many months past weaning her son, learned to her surprise how quickly milk can return.

Sharon: *My friend from Oregon came to visit us during a beautiful, snowy winter in Minnesota. My sons were five and a half and three and a half, at the ages where they loved sledding and building forts in the snow. Dawn's son, Morgan, was just four months old and preferred to stay inside and snuggle. I was more than happy to provide the arms for snuggling, while Dawn was content to bundle up and play in the snow with my sons. Morgan woke up while they were all outside and was root-ing at my breast. He had done that with me earlier and Dawn had said I could offer him my breast. I did just that and he snuggled right back down, content to be suckling (his mama had fed him not long before). I wasn't producing milk any longer, as my youngest had weaned several months earlier, so I was surprised when, after suckling off and on over a few hours, Morgan pulled away wide-eyed to look up at me and there was milk dribbling from both his mouth and my breast.*

To be able to make milk at all is a wonderful feeling. It's impressive—so much so that, after you wean your baby, you might even become curious to know if you can still express some milk from your breasts. I found that I could still do this more than twenty years after weaning my last child, and this is not unusual, as I've talked to more women than I can count who could do the same thing. Women in indigenous societies have, no doubt, experienced similar feelings, and they have the additional advantage of having grown up observing older women in their own villages nurse their grandchildren or adopted babies.

Of course, the baby has to be a willing participant in getting Granny's milk to start flowing again. In case anyone thinks that a baby might find Grandmother's breast too wrinkled to be attractive, think again. To babies, breasts are breasts, and they are not at all put off by the age of their owner. Babies love breasts, and they love them with absolutely no reservations, guilt, or shame.

It should be mentioned here that babies do recognize differences in the milk of their mother and that of another. As discussed earlier, the baby who is allowed to lick her mother's nipple during the few minutes after birth will be able to reliably distinguish her own mother's breast pad by smell from the breast pads of other mothers. Even with this ability to distinguish her own mother's milk, a hungry baby will nurse from "strange breasts." Some older babies or toddlers are adventurous in their tastes too. I remember one little boy of my acquaintance, whose full-breasted mother had nursed him for a year and a half. He had just turned two and was cuddled in his babysitter's lap, his face just even with the small breasts under her T-shirt.

"Is there any tits in that shirt?" he asked.

"Yes," she laughed, never having been asked such a thing before.

"Can I eat them?" he asked quietly.

Spontaneous Lactation

One day I was talking to a group of young women who were studying to be doulas, and I mentioned the ability of grandmothers to relactate. After the class, one of the women came up to me and said that she had had an interesting experience as a teenager that I might want to know about. It seems that she had been raised by a single mother and that she and her mother had often lived with other single mothers and their children. As the oldest child, this meant that she had a lot of contact with young babies as she was growing up. When she was fourteen or fifteen years old, she had a babysitting job for a couple of doctors with three children, one of whom was a very colicky baby about five months old. This young woman, Elizabeth, was extremely conscientious in how she cared for these children. On this particular day, she continued to hold the fussy baby in her arms over a period of hours, always trying to comfort him as she cared for the older children. Several hours had passed this way, without the baby quieting down for a nap. She was standing at the stove, still holding the baby and heating up some food for the older kids, when she felt a tingling sensation all over her body and a sudden wet feeling on her chest. She was astonished to see two wet circles forming on her T-shirt just over her small breasts, and the baby was diving toward them. Realizing that this was milk, she took the most practical approach she could to the situation and sat down in a comfortable chair, lifted her shirt, and allowed the baby to suckle. He gulped noisily for several minutes before falling into a deep sleep, satiated and blissful.

When the parents returned home, she told them what had happened. They had no problem with what she had done but were instead happy to know that their baby was sleeping and calm. Elizabeth told me that when her mother arrived to drive her home, she asked her to stop by a department store to buy a bra to help disguise how big her breasts had suddenly become. "I'm going to get such a hard time from the other kids," she told her mother. Elizabeth told me that her breasts were still full of milk until her period returned. She was twenty-five at the time she told me this story and said that she still felt the letdown reflex whenever she heard a baby cry and had to press on her breasts to keep them from secreting milk at such times.

Though not common, Elizabeth's experience was not unique to her. Returning to H. A. Wieschhoff's article, I found this reference to spontaneous lactation in the part of the article devoted to India: "...the Lepcha maintain that women who have never borne a child can produce milk which may be indigestible at first, but later becomes satisfactory." In addition, the superintendent in a hospital in Rajputana remarked that he had observed a Muslim woman, forty years old, "who had never borne children, nor had anything like an abortion in all her life. She was seen nursing her husband's grandchild by another woman and had done so for many months." According to the woman, the flow of milk was copious and was quite enough to satisfy the child.

Another young woman, Maria, told me of a similar experience she had—spontaneous lactation without ever having had a pregnancy. On impulse, I asked her if this experience involved a baby that she loved. Surprised, she answered that, yes, it did. She was living with her boyfriend, who had a six-month-old baby with a former girlfriend. The boyfriend was being allowed to care for the baby over the weekend for the first time. Maria, who was holding the baby while taking a warm shower, was surprised to notice milk spurting from each of her breasts.

Months later, at a routine gynecological examination, Maria was asked to fill out a form about her medical history. When she came to the question asking whether she had ever experienced a "discharge" from her breasts, she told me that she had answered yes—although she didn't really consider milk to be a discharge. To her surprise, the doctor ordered a CT scan, thinking that this symptom made it necessary to rule out a brain tumor. While spontaneous lactation can be a symptom of a brain tumor near the pituitary gland, it seems that most medical professionals no longer recognize that a healthy young woman with an extraordinary sympathy for babies can lactate spontaneously from nonpathological changes in her hormone levels.

Chloe's story illustrates how forgotten knowledge creates a narrowed view of women's bodies, so that phenomena that happen to especially sensitive women are seen as evidence of pathology. Only when women feel free to tell their stories can we begin to get an idea of the incidence of spontaneous, nonpathological lactation. My own sense is that it is much more common than we believe.

❧ **Chloe:** *In 2002, when I was twenty-two years old, I started working as a health-care assistant on a maternity unit while I was waiting for my nursing course to start. I've wanted to be a midwife since I can remember. It feels like something I was born to do, so when I started working at my local maternity unit, I just loved going to work. Mostly my duties consisted of breastfeeding support and general care of Mum and baby on the postnatal ward, with some occasional labor and birth support.*

A few months after being in this job, I was washing in the shower and noticed small amounts of yellow/white fluid at the end of my nipple. If I squeezed my breast to the end of my nipple, more would come, although not a lot. Having been providing breastfeeding support, I knew this fluid looked like colostrum or milk, and I was confused and concerned as to why this was happening. I asked my partner at the time if he had noticed anything, and he said that it was something he'd noticed recently but hadn't thought to mention it. I think the both of us were embarrassed; I know I was.

I made an appointment with my general practitioner (GP), who wanted to do a blood test, which I had, and when I returned for the results I had a high level of prolactin. When I asked my GP what was causing this, he was reluctant to enter into any discussion and referred me to an endocrinologist. When I saw this doctor, he told me that the rise in my hormone level could be due to a problem in my pituitary gland, which could be caused by a tumor. I was obviously extremely worried now, made worse by a long period of time where I had to wait to have an MRI, a bone scan to check my bone density, and an abdominal scan to check my ovaries. Nothing was found to be wrong, and the doctor was unable to tell me what was causing my prolactin level to be so high. Although relieved not to have a tumor, I was still made to feel there was something wrong, and I was also worried about the effects on my fertility. He gave me some medication, which I can't remember the name of, and I took this for three months with no change. I finally decided that I didn't want to be on any medication and I would leave things as they were. Having separated from my partner, I wasn't feeling embarrassed in front of anyone at present, and I pushed it to the back of my mind and got on with my nursing course.

I am now about to qualify as a midwife, and to this day I continue to lactate. It very rarely leaks from my nipples without some form of pressure applied to my breast, although there have been times during a birthing that it has. I have become very used to this and personally I don't really mind. However, it has stopped me being intimate with men, and I haven't had a relationship since—although I'm sure there are other reasons for this than just my lactation. I am still embarrassed, especially as when my breast is squeezed the milk can spurt out a lot. On a recent visit to The Farm, however, I met another woman who experiences this, who has a happy marriage and beautiful children. Ina May also suggested to me that it may not be such a coincidence that this began when I started my job, given that I love it so much and that I might *actually be experiencing higher levels of oxytocin, which, in turn, trigger the prolactin. Suddenly—and I can't believe I haven't made this connection myself—I feel like I'm not ill or weird but just highly sensitive to my job and the women I care for, and I wouldn't change the way I am for the world.*

Some of the best advice I got from my high school education was from my biology teacher, who told our class: "Always keep your mind open to new opportunities to learn." I continue trying to do that.

15

NIPPLEPHOBIA: WHAT IT IS AND WHY WE SHOULD ERADICATE IT

In the mid-1990s, I traveled to Oslo, Norway, to attend an international midwifery conference. At the time, I was publishing *Birth Gazette*, a quarterly magazine for midwives that focused on issues related to birth and breastfeeding. Always looking for advertisers, I was especially interested in teaching materials from other countries that might be good to promote back at home. As I strolled through the enormous exhibition hall, I came across a booth featuring a new Norwegian-made video about breastfeeding titled *Breast is Best*. What initially caught my attention was its cover: On the right, against a black background, was the profile of a nude breast, and on the left, a red rosebud just beginning to open. The idea behind this juxtaposition was that both the rosebud and the nipple are beautiful and tender. Intrigued, I sat down to view the video and found it the best I had seen, for several reasons. The information was accurate and well presented, but what I enjoyed most was the program's message that Norwegian women are able to nurse their babies without having to carry special clothing, shawls, giant bibs, or capes to cover themselves, as if they were doing something shameful that should be hidden. There they were, nursing their babies on crowded subways, in posh restaurants, in airport lounges, in parks—there seemed to be no restrictions at all on public breastfeeding.

Prior to my trip, over a period of fifteen years or so, women from all over the United States had been sending me news items about nursing mothers being told to leave cafés, restaurants, theaters, hotel lobbies, shopping malls, museums, and hotel or private membership swimming pools and to finish their feeding in the public toilet. (Babies are the only citizens of our country who can be sometimes required to eat in the bathroom—if their mothers can be bullied into going there.) To the business proprietors, managers, security police, and official personnel across the country who triggered these incidents, it didn't matter—and still doesn't, to many—that the American Academy of Pediatrics (AAP) had long recommended that all U.S. babies be exclusively breastfed for the first six months. It also didn't matter that in 1981, in an effort to boost rates of breastfeeding worldwide, the WHO/UNICEF Code of Marketing of Breast-Milk Substitutes was overwhelmingly approved by 118 countries in Geneva, Switzerland. What did count was that the United States was the *only* country in the world to vote against the WHO/UNICEF Code.

The WHO/UNICEF Code was a response to the millions of infant deaths worldwide that had ensued from substitute-milk companies' aggressive marketing campaigns. An international standard rather than a law, the code was a document that recommended that member governments restrict the advertising and sales promotions of breast-milk substitutes as a "minimum requirement" to protecting infant health. (See Appendix C for The Ten Steps to Successful Breastfeeding, one of the provisions of the code.) Voting for the code would not have restricted the availability or sale of breast-milk substitutes anywhere in the world. By voting for it, our country would have joined a worldwide effort to stop formula corporations from manipulating maternity-care services, which were promoting manufactured infant foods by sabotaging breastfeeding immediately following birth. By voting against the code, our federal government moved decisively to put the interests of the infant-formula corporations *ahead* of the health interests of mothers and babies in this country and the rest of the world. It may have been mere coincidence, but it was soon after the U.S. vote against the

WHO/UNICEF Code that incidents involving harassment of nursing mothers began to be reported by local television stations and newspapers across the country.

If only one way of infant feeding is permitted to be shown on television, in the movies, and on social networking sites on the Internet, that way of feeding, in effect, becomes something like a monopoly. If women are made to feel anxious about their breasts or ashamed of them, breastfeeding becomes a less likely option for them. Needed information about this way of feeding is effectively blocked in the public media on the false basis of "modesty." The choice for many is narrowed to which brand of infant formula to buy and what kind of bottle to put it in. Consider, for instance, how the symbol of the bottle has become the metaphor for infant feeding in the public media of cartoons, magazines, children's books, and movies; there is little federal effort to counter the impression that bottle-feeding of artificial milks is better, more reliable, and more socially acceptable than breastfeeding for a human infant.

The pattern set at the federal level in 1981 has changed very little in the years since. The Department of Health and Human Services set a national goal for 2010 for half of all U.S. mothers to be still breastfeeding when their babies are six months old. At the time of this writing, less than twenty-nine percent are still breastfeeding at six months, while eighty percent of Norwegian babies are still getting their mothers' milk at that time. The question arises: Why have a goal if there is no national strategy to reach it? It's a sure recipe for frustration and backlash against breastfeeding when a government states goals for breastfeeding women but provides little information or legislative support to make such goals attainable.

Some people (there is no way to quantify how many) in our society apparently think that nursing mothers should never leave their homes with their babies until they are weaned. They obviously aren't thinking about what it would be like to be a mother or a baby under these conditions. In the nineteenth century and earlier, it was customary for U.S. women to stay home most of the time when they had young babies; in fact, this period was even called "confinement." Today, such isolation is close to impossible for anyone who isn't already a hermit or who has other children. Mothers in some parts of the United States were and sometimes still are treated like naughty children, being banished to a public toilet stall if they insist on continuing their feeding—some are harassed even when they have done everything possible to occupy their "own space" while out and about. I remember, for instance, the Missouri mother who was ticketed for "indecent exposure" for nursing her baby in her car in a far corner of a shopping-mall parking lot in the 1980s. In another instance, in 2007, a Madison, Wisconsin, mother was feeding her young baby in her car in a mall parking lot when she was interrupted by a security guard tapping on her window, telling her, "You can't do that here."

In many European countries—Austria, Norway, Sweden, Germany, Denmark, Italy, and Iceland are examples where I've been recently—public spaces such as malls, department stores, airports, train stations, and museums provide attractive, comfortable places for nursing mothers and their babies to sit down for a feed. There is often a choice between a private place (where a woman might need to pump her milk) or an area that is designated for families with a nursing baby and older siblings (where breastfeeding is as acceptable as bottle-feeding). In the United States, on the other hand, it is far less likely for public places to take into account the needs of women who nurse their babies. I was recently in an airport in the nation's capital, in which the designated "lactation room" offered only one hard bench, with no sink for washing hands and no place that would accommodate an older child. This room was separated by only a thin wall from the public toilet stalls with their constant flushing.

Although more U.S. women are nursing their babies during the first few weeks of life than a generation ago and progress has been made during that time (about half of the states have passed some sort of law meant to protect the rights of nursing mothers), harassment still does occur, most likely because states don't yet have laws that penalize the act of harassing a nursing mother. Laws should provide for penalties when they are broken. It's about time that our legislatures—state and federal—protect the needs of nursing mothers and their babies for a change.

One of the best-known U.S. writers on etiquette over the last quarter century, Judith Martin (aka "Miss Manners"), offered the opinion in one of her books that nursing mothers should never feed their babies in a room—even in their own homes—where other people are present. "The argument that it is a natural function carries no weight whatsoever," she wrote. "Would you change the baby's diaper on the dining-room table while people are eating? That's also a natural function." I would say that Miss Manners got the ends of the baby mixed up, not to mention the difference between food and feces. Despite all the information that's available to literate people in breastfeeding books and on the Internet, she has never seen fit to retract her bent opinion that breastfeeding is in bad taste.

It's possible that Miss Manners was helped to form her strong opinion on breastfeeding by a campaign begun in the early 1970s by a media prankster named Alan Abel. One of Abel's earlier campaigns—his Society for Indecency to Naked Animals (SINA)—had already gained widespread media exposure, as it lobbied for the passage of laws requiring all animals to wear clothing to cover their genitals (in order to wipe out the double standard between humans and animals regarding what was considered indecent). Abel argued his absurd case on *The Tonight Show,* the *Today* show, and even *The CBS Evening News with Walter Cronkite* before revealing that it was all a hoax. His campaign to make breastfeeding illegal by claiming that it was perverse, incestuous, and led to homosexuality and "oral fixations" such as smoking and drinking later in life was a similarly absurd attempt to spoof U.S. puritanical attitudes related to the body. It, too, received remarkable media coverage. The trouble was that, instead of laughter and disbelief, it provoked anger and indignation on the part of people who didn't recognize it as an elaborate media hoax. Weirdly, Abel's rhetoric, once adopted and popularized by Miss Manners, became common in the debates surrounding public breastfeeding, and things he said in jest are now put forward with all seriousness—sometimes even by women who have breastfed.

At any rate, there I was in Oslo in the mid-1990s, feeling quite fascinated with Norway's accommodations for nursing mothers. I sat down to talk with Gudrun Stie, the producer of *Breast is Best.* She told me that in the early 1970s, Norway had rates of breastfeeding as low as those in the United States (about a fifth of women nursed their babies for the first few weeks, and hardly anyone continued through the first year) but now Norway led the world in rates of breastfeeding through babies' first year of life. I wanted to understand how Norway had accomplished such a drastic social change so rapidly. It turns out that the United States had provided the initial inspiration through La Leche League's book *The Womanly Art of Breastfeeding.* A Norwegian woman who had read the book sometime during the late 1960s was so impressed to learn about the enormous health benefits of nursing that she contacted Norway's health minister about what could be done to increase the number of Norwegian babies getting mother's milk. At that time, Gro Harlem Brundtland, a family physician with a master's degree in public health from Harvard (who had written her thesis on declining rates of breastfeeding), was working in Norway's Directorate of Health. A little more than a decade later, Brundtland was elected Norway's first woman prime minister and spent about a decade in that post during the 1980s and 1990s, later serving as director-general of the World Health Organization. During part of her time as prime minister, with eight women among her eighteen cabinet ministers and a sizable proportion of women in Parliament—Norway passed a law requiring that every hospital in the country be "Baby-Friendly." That ended any marketing influence that infant-formula companies had formerly wielded in Norway's hospitals. Rooming-in became the norm instead of the exception, and hospital staff were retrained in how to facilitate rather than sabotage (however unintentionally) the initiation of breast-feeding during mothers' and babies' stays in hospital.

It was impossible for me not to notice that the women's movement in Norway during the 1960s and 1970s took a different, more inclusive course from that taken in the United States during the same period. The main goals of feminist leaders here focused on making it possible (and safer) for women to choose *not* to be mothers, expanding women's access to higher education and jobs and professions that had previously been closed to them, giving women the means to combat sexual harassment and domestic violence, and creating access to political office. Norway's feminists worked on all of these issues but on another vitally important area as well: *They demanded legislation that would significantly benefit Norwegian mothers and babies.* Paid maternity leave, on-site nursery care in the workplace, flexible schedules for working women, and parental benefits were all part of the legislative advances made in Norway during the 1960s and 1970s. Architects followed suit by designing shopping malls, airports, and other public areas with comfortable, attractive places for nursing women and their children to use.

Another part of my conversation with Gudrun Stie concerned the visual message of *Breast is Best.* With an undraped breast with nipple as the main design element on the video cover, she had discovered that distributors in some countries were stipulating that they must have permission to change the cover design to one that didn't show a nipple

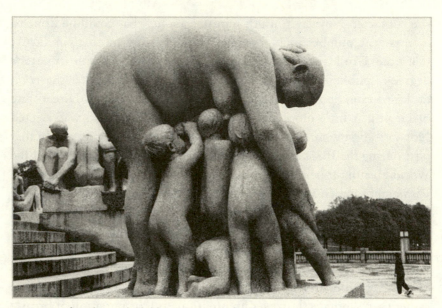

Statue of mother with children in Vigeland's Sculpture Park

or areola if they were to sell her product. Despite the potential setback this might mean for marketing her video, she refused to change the cover design, because she and her production team strongly believed that the cover conveyed an essential part of the program's message. This was their argument: "If a country is going to get serious about increasing rates of breastfeeding, people are going to have to get used to seeing nipples sometimes." I couldn't have agreed more.

On my return trip from Oslo, I was full of ideas about how to make life easier for nursing mothers and their babies back home. I began to understand that Norway's success in resuscitating this primal feminine art had been possible not only because of bold action at the political and legislative level but also because Norway's culture had been more able than ours to accept the presence of babies and their needs among us. Even though Norwegians during the 1970s, like North Americans, had had little chance to see nursing mothers for some decades, people there had somehow adapted to and accepted the sight and sounds of a mother nursing her baby wherever women might want or need to be. Too many North Americans hadn't.

I had taken this first trip to Norway anticipating that modern-day Norwegians might remind me of the repressed people in Henrik Ibsen's plays or the somber Norwegian American farmers I knew from my childhood in Iowa (especially the one who always slept in the barn rather than in the house with his wife and whose only entertainment, according to my parents, was going to girls' basketball games and Norwegian funerals). What I found in Oslo was quite different from my expectations. In fact, modern-day Norwegians seemed to me far less repressed than many of the people back in the United States.

Flying home, I began to wonder how much the work of the amazing sculptor Gustav Vigeland had to do with Norway's ability to successfully promote breastfeeding in everyday culture. My mind was full of vivid memories of the afternoon I had spent wandering around Vigeland's Sculpture Park on the outskirts of Oslo. Vigeland worked for the last two decades of his life on this mammoth project, which occupies eighty acres and includes more than two hundred bronze or granite sculptures of nude people in all stages of life. The park was opened to the public in 1947, about four years after the sculptor's death. Collected in thirty-six different groups, the sculptures have an emotional reality that is rare in this art form. Each is so expressive that it seems to be alive. There are neither drapes nor fig leaves, and there's nothing coy about

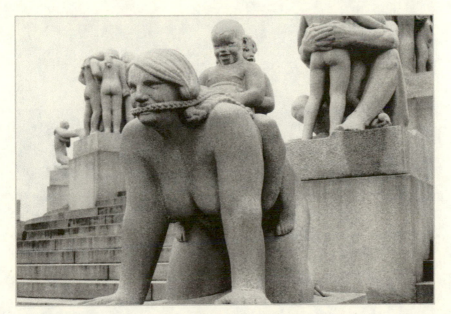

Mother playing "horsey" with children in Vigeland's Sculpture Park

any of the figures—no hands shielding the breasts or crotch. The nudity is more matter-of-fact than defiant and certainly adds a dimension of vulnerability. Each sculpture conveys the feeling that the figures themselves don't realize that they are nude, any more than a bear or horse would. Instead, they all seem to be alive and feeling some emotion that is strongly evoked in facial and bodily expression or a captured moment of powerful movement.

My feeling is that Vigeland created his immense project at least in part to show people how to relate in kindly ways to one another in whatever relationships occur between people of different ages and genders. Vigeland himself felt that the meaning of his work was so clear that even a child might understand it. The several children in the park on the day I was there appeared to have been there before, and they had their favorites. They climbed on laps or backs of some of the figures (as, I am sure, they were meant to).

Late in his life, Vigeland remarked, "West Norwegian Puritanism contains a vast fund of emotion. When it is turned in another direction, when it follows another course, then it has enormous power and can accomplish great things."

Probably more than anything, I wished that such a park existed in the

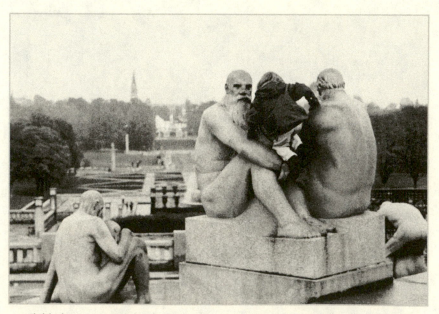

Child playing on Vigeland sculpture

United States, because I felt sure that Vigeland's sculptures were at least part of the reason that the portion of the Norwegian public that wasn't used to public breastfeeding was able to accept the needs of nursing babies to eat wherever their mothers might be. It is likely that most every Norwegian adult during the 1970s and thereafter has spent several hours as a child playing among the groups of figures in the park. The healthy sexuality that is evident in Vigeland's work has been called "the strongest blow that has ever been struck against pornography in art, because it represents the rational expression of sexuality." Although this great artist is not very well known outside of Norway and isn't generally to be found in art-history books, I found his Sculpture Park to be one of the most profound works I have ever had the privilege to see. I kept thinking of him as one who had the unusual gift of depicting emotion and human sensuality in a very pure and healing way. Could we in the United States permit an artist to do what he did in Oslo? How about in Minnesota?

On that flight home, I began to think more deeply about the set of attitudes and behaviors that gets between babies and their food as a manifestation of a severe mental disorder that has taken hold and become widespread across the North American continent. In what species besides our own would adult males or females harass a mother in the act of nourishing her young? Such behavior would not occur to any other creature. What makes this behavior seem downright crazy to me is that even people who love the baby can be uncompassionate enough to disrupt dinner by being unpleasant to both mother and baby at a time when they are vulnerable. I'm thinking now of the IBM "Milk Mom," who wrote in the delightful book *Milk Memos* of her visit to her mother-in-law's Kansas home with her three-month-old nursing baby. On the first day of vacation, she sat in the living room, having a quiet nursing moment with him. Suddenly, Grandmother appeared and threw an old brown afghan over both of them (in a room that was already heated to seventy-five degrees). The baby cried and "yanked it down as fast as I could pull it up on my shoulder. And that was just day one!" wrote the mother.

The grandmother in this case surely loved her grandson but couldn't stop herself from being unpleasant to him as he was eating. This wasn't "Would you like a blanket, dear?" It was unilateral action without explanation or apology—a kind of punishment, really. I find this kind of behavior neurotic at best, but when it represents the norm for millions of people, I think we have reached the realm of near-psychosis—mass mental illness. If we humans watched adult birds diving and pecking at mother birds as they attempted to stuff worms and insects into the gaping beaks of their chicks, we would think we were watching a horror movie about birds gone mad. It *is* horrible to see adults behaving in an infantile way that doesn't nurture the generations to come.

Recently, a nursing-mom blogger remarked on longtime media personality Barbara Walters's comment on a popular women's morning television show that she had been made uncomfortable and "very nervous" on a flight from London because a woman in a seat across the aisle had nursed her baby, and "she didn't cover the baby with a blanket." Mind you: This was first-class seating—Barbara Walters doesn't fly economy. What did she expect the baby to eat and what did she expect the mother to do about her overfull breasts?

For the blogger, the real issue had less to do with the comfort of fellow passengers and more to do with the baby: "As a nursing mother, my take on the situation is fairly personal. I'm offended at the unaccountable offense. When I nurse my child, I do so for her. Her comfort and hunger are the first priority. The next priority is my comfort while carrying out the task. The last thing I worry about, or should worry about, is someone attempting to sexualize (which is where the squeamishness comes from) the tool I use to feed my child.

"Additionally, the ignorance about how important nursing on airplanes is for the child is unexpected from a woman reportedly as intelligent as Walters. When it comes to protecting my child's eardrums from rupturing, or even discomfort, my child is always going to come first. (When she wouldn't nurse on the plane when we visited my folks at Christmas, the result was a 102.5 temperature and a trip to the emergency room.)"

U.S. squeamishness about breasts being used for their biological purpose dates back at least to the Civil War period. People who were enthralled by what seemed to them a new scientific approach to life and the promise of technology invented ways to feed babies without having direct contact with their mothers' breasts. Some of the contraptions were bottle-holding devices that would allow a mother to prop her hungry baby, who would then drink from a rubber nipple and tube leading to the bottle while the mother did something else. In 1910, an "anti-embarrassment device"—a leather bra with heavy metal buckles, a rubber nipple, and long tubing that was to be worn by nursing mothers when they had to be in public—was granted a patent by the U.S. Patent Office. The ad for this bizarre creation showed a drawing of a woman wearing the device (which was drawn in loving detail, in contrast with the dotted lines suggesting her form and that of the baby) while holding a baby sprawled on her lap. A long tube led from the rubber or leather circle that covered her nipples to the rubber nipple that the baby was meant to suck.

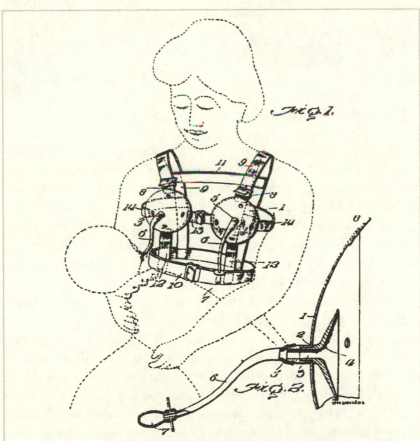

This nursing attachment was "designed to avoid unpleasant and embarrassing situations in which mothers are sometimes placed in public places by the necessary exposure of the breast in suckling." *Courtesy*: U.S. Patent Office, Patent No. 949414, 1910. Patented by Hugh Cunningham.

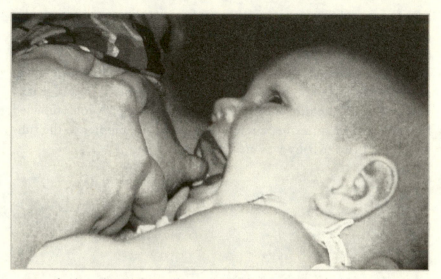
Breastfeeding photo that was deemed "obscene" by Walmart

No one knows how many people actually used the "nursing attachment," as it was called, but public-health nurses around that time found it necessary to issue warnings to mothers that feeding devices that used any kind of rubber tubes were "baby killers," because they were impossible to keep clean. "Cut the tube open, smell it, and see!" one poster warned. The people who promoted and bought such devices accepted the belief that babies need nothing beyond the bare physical necessities of food, sleep, warmth, and protection against illness.

The same bent imagination that led an inventor to create the "anti-embarrassment device" seems to have invaded the photo-printing departments of some U.S. chain stores. Andie Wyrick, a young Texas mother, dropped off some photos for developing at a Walmart store in 2006. When she returned to pick them up, she found all but one in the envelope. In place of the missing photo, she found a piece of paper that said, "Walmart has found one or more of your photographs to be of an inappropriate and/or obscene nature." The photo in question was of her three-month-old daughter happily gaping to receive her mother's breast.

🌿 **Andie:** *How could someone find a normal, natural, and beautiful photograph obscene? I wrestled with the urge to question Walmart and finally decided it was important to follow through. I talked to associates*

inside and outside of the photo department, both female and male. I spoke to employees and managers galore. I even talked to the ethics line but was told they could only help employees. Communication consisted of emails and phone calls. Initially, no one had answers. I got robotic apologies such as, "We're so sorry for your frustration, but it's our policy and it's up to each employee." Once they even asked, "Does it show your nipple and that colored areola thing?" They said skin is okay, but nipples are blatant. I would say, "Okay, is there any way I can get that policy in writing, so I can read it?" This is when I found out that a policy didn't actually exist. They told me as they were getting backed into the corner that it was "just known—the same way it's known that you can't slap a customer in the face." My persistence, although annoying to Walmart, ended with an understanding, at least at the location that I frequent. They had a storewide meeting about my photograph and the rules of developing "obscene" pictures. They concluded that breastfeeding photographs should not be grouped with pictures deemed obscene and inappropriate like those of a sexual nature, penetration, child pornography, and blatant nudity any longer. I couldn't believe my nursing infant was ever classified with child pornography or sex. How could someone see that photo through those kinds of eyes? My innocent baby captured while eating caused all this commotion. It's hard to continue what you know is right and perfect for your child when the world gives you such a battle.

A popular parenting magazine, *BabyTalk,* ran a cover in the summer of 2006 featuring a photo of a nursing baby. This particular issue focused especially on breastfeeding. All that was visible was a smiling baby's face and the side view of her mother's breast (with no nipple showing). A flood of letters poured in—more than had come in response to any other article in the magazine's history. The editors polled their readers, and more than a quarter of them called the photo "inappropriate." A sampling of their comments included the following, which tellingly reveal the angst and confusion that surrounds many women's attitudes toward women's bodies:

- "I was SHOCKED to see a giant breast on the cover of your magazine."

- "I immediately turned the magazine facedown."

- "Gross."

- "I shredded it," said a Texas woman. "A breast is a breast—it's a sexual thing. My thirteen-year-old son didn't need to see that."

- "I don't want my son or husband to accidentally see a breast they didn't want to see."

According to *BabyTalk*'s editor, Susan Kane, "There's a huge puritanical streak in Americans, and there's a squeamishness about seeing a body part—even part of a body part. It's not like women are whipping them out with tassels on them! Mostly, they are trying to be discreet."

Facebook, the popular social-networking site, came down on the side of extreme puritanism in 2008 when it banned its members from putting breastfeeding photos into their profiles. Within a few days, more than 100,000 members had signed a petition titled "Hey, Facebook, breastfeeding is not obscene!"

People who are uncomfortable with breastfeeding don't realize that when breasts can't be seen performing their intended function, people reach the absurd condition of not knowing what the intended function is. Could any species other than the human have an external organ and not know what it was for?

Truly, we are talking about a kind of cultural madness. Here we are taught to think of the British as the most puritanical culture possible regarding female nudity,

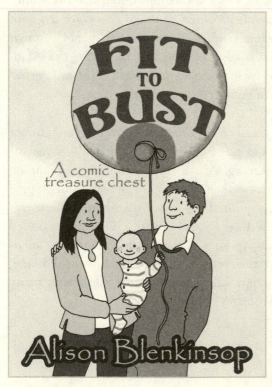

Fit to Bust cover

but our standards are far more restrictive than the Brits'. It's possible, for instance, for a British book cover to feature a visual joke like that featured on Alison Blenkinsop's book *Fit to Bust,* published in 2008 in the U.K.

When she asked me if it would be possible to publish a U.S. edition of her book, I had to tell her that it probably wouldn't—at least, not with that cover. Having seen for myself that it is possible for adult humans to behave rationally and kindly to mothers and babies (my community and Norway are just two examples of many that can be found around the world), I'm urging us to find a cure for what ails U.S. society in this regard. The title of Japanese novelist Kenzaburo Oe's short novel seems apropos: *Teach Us to Outgrow Our Madness.*

Maria Lactans

There is a long, rich history in Christian art of depicting the madonna as a lactating mother. The genre is called "Maria Lactans" by art historians (Latin for "Mary lactating"). The first known work in this genre was finished in approximately 250 A.D., and artists continued to reimagine this theme over the next fifteen centuries. I have never seen a painting of baby Jesus being bottle-fed, although I wouldn't be surprised if one has been created by this time. If someone did fashion such a work, many in my country might find nothing historically wrong with it. What I suspect *would* surprise most people in my country is that in the many paintings and sculptures of Mary nursing

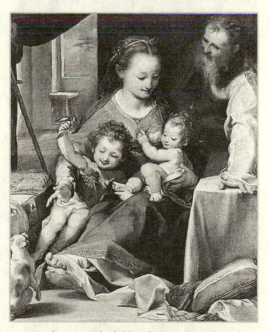

"Madonna and Child with Saint Joseph and the Infant Baptist" by Federico Barocci required no drapes over the Madonna's breast to qualify as a sacred painting.

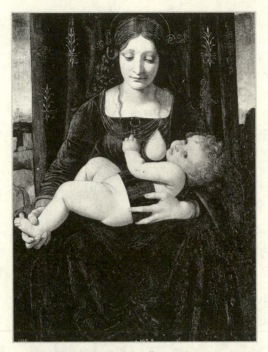

Giovanni Antonio Boltraffio's "The Virgin and Child" depicts the sacred relationship for an altarpiece. Many paintings of this kind feature the Child as a large toddler.

Jesus, the artists never considered it disrespectful to Jesus or Mary to show her breast and nipple. Sometimes these paintings depict a baby Jesus who is temporarily distracted by the sight of another child, so Mary's breast is left exposed as she tries to entice him to finish the feeding.

Is there a copy of a Maria Lactans in any church in the United States? Apart from one such work of art venerated at the Shrine of Our Lady of La Leche in St. Augustine, Florida, and perhaps some old churches in New Mexico (my husband remembers seeing one in Santa Fe), I know of no other.

I found an interesting discussion on the subject of whether or not a breastfeeding mother should attend a worship service on the website of Rev. Dr. Renita J. Weems, an African American preacher–theologian who has a popular and well-written blog (www.somethingwithin.com). A woman who clearly prides herself on her willingness to buck church authority and poke holes in religious orthodoxy, she found herself questioning her own iconoclasm in November 2007, when this subject came up. It seems that during Rev. Weems's sermon, an usher went over and told a young mother with a baby at her breast that such behavior wasn't allowed in a church with this particular congregation, which was largely African American. The embarrassed mother gathered up her things and her squalling baby as they were ushered out of the "sanctuary." By the time the baby was done nursing, the sermon was over and it was offering time. Rev. Weems went on to lead a discussion of how to reconcile strong women's views on gender equality, gender discrimination, sexually degrading images of black women in the media, and violence against women with the message to this young mother that she wasn't welcome in church. One woman wrote: "The idea of a child learning from infancy to associate the comfort of Mom with the comfort of God (being fed during the sermon) seems ideal to me. Would not The Breasted One want such an association?" (The Breasted One is a translation of the divine name *El Shaddai*, Rev. Weems instructed her readers.) Another woman, a preacher herself, responded this way: "Prior to having a child I would have been much more conscious of where, when and in front of whom I would whip out my breast. However, in light of the overwhelming responsibility of caring for a newborn (at least from my perspective), I have become more lax and when my baby girl cries, I don't care who's around to see. My brother-in-law has even become more familiar with me than he ever thought he would. As one who still gets a little nervous because of the embarrassment that might occur at the sound of my wailing baby, I find no harm in tending to her needs in public, including church. I must admit, I am a bit clumsy with those nursing covers that don't quite cover when you're a healthy well-endowed woman, if you know what I mean. They always seem to get in the way and make my baby sweat something awful. Recently, when I was preaching, a friend of mine whipped out her breast and began to feed her son. Yes, she was covered. I thought it was phenomenal that she was able to do such so unassumingly. Indeed, I think the church has some learning to do in this area. Indeed, we have become too westernized with many of our preferences. I agree that much of this is centered around our thoughts about the black female body. Will we never escape the gaze even from our own sisters? When our foremothers nursed entire communities, do you think they did so in shame? In some ways, asking women to cover perpetuates the shame that often accompanies black women's feelings about their bodies."

Feelings of shame and revulsion are foreign in many cultures, if not in our own. An old gentleman who lived at The Farm until his death a few years ago told me a great story about an incident he remembered from his life in Belgium before World War II.

"When I lived in Antwerp, I used to follow crowds to the zoo. In my opinion, these people knew how to relax and enjoy themselves. After you had viewed all the animals and marveled at all the beautiful flowers, you would go to the beer garden and order sandwiches and beer. All day long, there would be bands. It was the perfect way to spend a day. One day while I was listening to the music, a baby started to cry, cry, cry. It was disturbing the music, until quite a bunch of people started to clap their hands in time with the music. They all started to yell, 'Titah! Titah! Titah!' The young mother started to laugh and began to nurse her child. Then she got a big hand for quieting the baby. I noticed that in Europe, no one gets excited when a woman nurses her child." Quite possibly, the lack of excitement about public nursing in Europe, compared with North America, has much to do with the tradition of Maria Lactans.

Here's my question: Is it possible that a major art gallery in New York City or Washington, D.C., could have a show of the many works showing baby Jesus breastfeeding? Maybe there should be a traveling show. Would this help cure North Americans of their breast fetish disorder? I suspect that it might help.

Naming the Disease

Since I hardly hold the power or position to arrange for portraits of baby Jesus nursing to be viewed by people of all ages in this vast country, I have to think of other ways to approach the problem of helping the people of my country to outgrow their madness. It occurs to me that the first step is to convince them that they do suffer from a mental disorder.

How can we discuss this public-health problem intelligently, let alone treat it, if it isn't named? I suggest that we call this mental disorder a phobia. Since this particular phobia focuses on nipples, we should probably just call it "nipplephobia." Somehow, that makes me feel better already.

Definition: irrational fear, fascination, attraction, repulsion, guilt, and confusion provoked by seeing an adult female nipple (or even the illusion that one is seeing one). Janet Jackson's famous "wardrobe malfunction" in 2004 caused a major television network to be fined a half million dollars by the Federal Communications Commission because, during a song-and-dance number, her male partner grabbed a flap on her leather jacket, supposedly exposing her nipple. Curious about the incident, which I hadn't witnessed live, I went to the Internet and found out that it wasn't really her nipple that was exposed but rather an elaborate piece of jewelry—a kind of sunburst—that was fixed to her pierced nipple. The incident dominated the news in this country for several days, while people in the rest of the world wondered what was wrong with us.

Most people in the United States have been taught by direct advertising campaigns to believe that the only ways to treat illnesses are with pharmaceutical drugs or with surgery. Happily, nipplephobia can be successfully treated without such drastic, expensive, and potentially risky means. All that is needed is visual-stimulus overload. Translation: Sufferers need to see more adult female nipples in a context that is not specifically sexual. When they reach overload, the symptoms of discomfort subside and normal life continues. Nipplephobes suffer from not having seen enough nipples during infancy and childhood. The frustration that results from this causes the reconceptualization of the breast as purely an organ of sexual attraction. In order to maintain this concept in full force, babies must not be seen near breasts, no matter how much they need them. The people who buy into this notion, whether male or female, tend to be upset and confused by the idea that the primary function of the breasts is for nurturing the young. At the same time, they tend to be unaware of the cost of this attitude to the babies who are denied the breast. For them, breasts are sexual organs and nothing else. As a counterpoint to this formulation, it is interesting to note that there are other cultures in which the view of breasts as sexual equipment would be seen as bizarre.

A male friend of mine, who had a chance to live in the Sinai Desert with a group of Bedouins during the 1960s, described the following experience.

"The Bedouins are a proud people who show a lot of love and respect for one another. They have a strong set of values and traditions. One tradition says that women must keep their faces veiled. This was different from anything I had ever lived around before, but what really had an effect on me was the time when one of these Bedouin women raised her robes, exposing her breasts to me as she fed her baby. She acted as if everything was perfectly all right. It was only I who was taken by surprise. I realized that in cultures in which women breastfeed their babies, everyone in that culture grows up seeing breasts being used as they are meant to be. They have a natural attitude toward them. It's only in cultures like ours, where you almost never see a woman breastfeeding, that

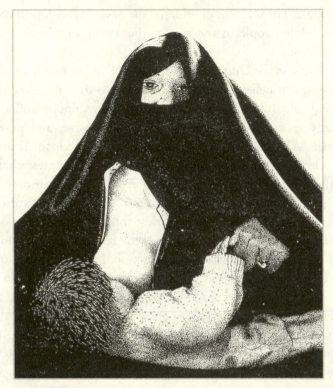

Muslim cultures value breastfeeding too highly to restrict babies' access to mothers' breasts.

breasts become the object for something else, usually something to lust after."

What my friend realized from this experience was the degree to which his own culture had created a concept of the female breast as fetish—in the psychiatric sense that a body part (or piece of clothing) sometimes becomes imbued with the power to arouse erotic feelings. Among the Bedouin, every part of a woman has this significance except for her breasts and, possibly, her hands! No wonder my friend was confused at first.

My friend's observation is corroborated by a Canadian woman of French Algerian ancestry, who wrote the following:

Farah: *This is the account of my grandmother's culture shock the first time she visited Algeria. She is a French woman who married an Arab man, my grandpa.*

What most struck her on that first visit to a Muslim country was the dress of the women. In Algeria, they robe themselves in long veils to guard their modesty, leaving only their eyes, hands, and feet exposed.

On a train ride between two cities, she saw such a woman wrapped in white drapes, except that one of those drapes was pulled up, thus allowing her breasts to be exposed, to the great satisfaction of a baby suckling from them.

In my grandmother's homeland, France, the opposite was true: Women showed their hair, their faces, their arms, and their legs without any embarrassments, but they never exposed their breasts—especially not their nipples—not even for the sake of a baby.

Though modesty of wear is compulsory in Islam, breastfeeding is also a religious obligation. It is even stated in the Holy Koran: *Mothers shall suckle their children for two whole years; (that is) for those who wish to complete the suckling term (Chapter 2, Verse 233).*

I know that visual-stimulus overload is the single most effective way to deal with nipplephobia, since that is how we dealt with this situation within The Farm community. It would have been unthinkable for anyone to tell a nursing mother to get out of their sight in our community, no matter how much nipple she showed before her baby latched on. If we nursing mothers made anyone uncomfortable, *they* were the ones who had to get over it. The best part was that they did. What men learned when they visited or joined our community (many had obviously never been around nursing mothers before) was that while it was okay to look, it was not all right to stare. At the same time, though, honesty requires me to report that just before I mailed this manuscript to my publisher, I learned that for the first time in the history of The Farm, a nursing mother was told (in this case, by a young lifeguard who, ironically, had himself been nursed at this swimming hole as an infant) that she would need to cover her baby with a towel if she was going to continue to nurse. She refused, and the young man quickly learned that the women in our community weren't willing to change to a more restrictive standard than that which had prevailed for decades. Nevertheless, this incident illustrates how contagious nipplephobia can be, since it can even affect those who weren't deprived of nursing as infants.

People who are nipplephobic need to realize that the burden is upon them to deal with their disease. They are just going to have to look at babies nursing and deal with whatever sexual images or feelings of jealousy or disgust come to mind when they see this happening. Buddhists know how to do this. Record the phenomena, but don't get hung up over whatever weird thoughts may come up. These will pass, like the thoughts that went before them. Gradually one gets better, and these weird thoughts will fade away. Laughter, of course, helps.

Dealing with Nipplephobia as a Nursing Mother

Those who intend to feed their babies nature's prescribed food will naturally want to know how they can navigate in a society whose medical experts extol the virtues of breastfeeding but whose social mores make little or no room for the act that accomplishes it. First, don't assume that you will meet with criticism if you choose to feed your baby the way nature intended wherever you happen to be. Even though you may have encountered several news stories of women who were asked to leave public places because they were feeding their babies, it's important to remember that most people will not harass you when you go out in public with your nursing baby. Yes, you may notice that people look at you longer than usual when they notice your baby is at your breast, but at least half of these people will probably approve of what you are doing. Some of them may even tell you so.

When you are going out into public for the first time with your nursing baby and feel nervous about it, consider taking a friend along with you. You might just have a positive experience something like the women whose stories are told below.

❧ **Faith:** *I was very modest and concerned about reaction to public breastfeeding with my first child—so much so that I would routinely pump breast milk and bring bottles to any outings in public so as not to be put in the position of having to breastfeed her in public. I had carefully learned all the "comfortable" bathrooms (ones with couches and lounges) and the stores that had lactation rooms or nursing rooms.*

When my daughter was six months old, we were having dinner at a chain restaurant near my home with extended family in for a visit. I had already fed my daughter (who was not on solids yet) the entire

supply of bottled breast milk I had with me, and she was still looking to nurse. I knew the bathrooms were single-stall not-very-clean toilets and therefore not an option. After trying to settle her down for a few minutes, I finally reconciled myself to the fact I would need to somehow discreetly nurse her in public, in the middle of a busy Friday-night dinner rush in a suburban restaurant. I opened my blouse and nursing bra and placed a napkin over my breast and child (who was now fussing and starting to cry). She was having trouble latching on and fussing even more, when all of a sudden, in one swift move, she grabbed the napkin, threw it off both of us, pulled off my breast, and let out this loud, angry scream.

Here I was, in the middle of this restaurant, breast fully exposed and everyone turning to look at me. And somehow, no one gawked or pointed or said anything negative—or anything at all. They just turned back to their conversations, my daughter latched on and nursed comfortably, and I never was uncomfortable again.

Melinda: *As I was sitting on a bench in the middle of the mall, alone, breastfeeding my infant daughter, two young men (probably sixteen to eighteen years old) strutted toward me in their loose, baggy jeans and T-shirts. I was very afraid of what they were going to say to me. I almost felt as if I wanted to get up and leave as they approached, being pretty sure they were going to harass me. As they came closer, one of them smiled and said to the other, as he pointed, "Hey, man, she's breastfeeding. That's so cool!"*

I could sense that he really meant it, and a sense of relief washed over me. I also felt a release of a stereotype I had held about teenage males. What a positive experience for both of us!

Colleen: *When Trudy, my first baby, was about six weeks old, my husband's grandfather came to visit. He is a history professor in his early nineties and had made the trip halfway across the country to visit. I was a new mom and didn't know much about what I was doing, but I held Trudy in my arms or a sling most of the time (except when she was being passed around the relatives) and nursed her whenever and wherever she wanted. At one point, toward the end of his stay, I got a little nervous when I saw Christopher turn toward me as I was feeding Trudy. He*

said, *"You know, I have to tell you, it is so beautiful to see you hold her and feed her like that." Such a lovely and welcome surprise!*

This also happened a few times in public with strangers—usually older women would be looking at us nursing. I'd start to feel nervous, but eventually they would come over and commend me for doing the right thing for my child. I am grateful to those people.

When you do face criticism, know that you don't need to take it. You are not doing anything wrong, so you should not let anyone make you feel otherwise. Here are stories from two mothers who came up with different ways of dealing with criticism they received for nursing in public:

Natasha: *I always feel like I'm doing people a favor when I nurse in public, because that's better than everyone having to listen to my baby crying. Crying is a very distressing sound for most people.*

Our recent Florida vacation was cut short, so we decided to pamper ourselves the last two days by staying at the Hilton in Orlando. I was at the pool with my five-month-old daughter, Penny, and my five-year-old son. I had hired a babysitter to hold Penny while she was sleeping. When she woke up after a long nap, of course she wanted to nurse, so I sat down and started nursing her, as I continued to watch my son swim. After a few minutes had passed, a bartender approached me and said that it was hotel policy that I should cover Penny up with a towel. Now, this was a really hot day, and we were already in the shade. There was no way that we could be comfortable doing that.

I said that I absolutely would not do that. I had intended to bring my copy of Mothering *magazine that contained an article about the legal status of nursing in public, in each of the states, but in my haste I had brought the wrong copy. However, I was pretty sure that there must be some federal legal protection covering such a situation, so I told her that I had the federally protected right to breastfeed wherever I happened to be. I said that it would be fine with me if she would like her manager to come out to talk to me. I continued feeding Penny, but I felt upset at being harassed, as we had come there to be pampered and I had already nursed in various parts of this hotel several times during our stay.*

When I finished nursing, I found that I was still bothered about having been harassed, especially since the manager apparently hadn't had the nerve to come and talk to me. I went to talk to the concierge and told her about my experience. She apologized profusely and then gave me her email address so that I could send her the law that I had mentioned.

I went up to my room and started getting upset about this again. I realized that I didn't have any confidence that the concierge would relay the problem I had to a level where something would be done about it. I realized that she had tried to appease me and, furthermore, that she had given me a task to do. I picked up Penny (who wanted to nurse again) and went down once more, and said, "I think the only way I am going to feel better about this situation is if I have an apology from the bartender who spoke with me and from her manager who sent her to do this."

"Okay, I'll go get them," she said. "Please wait."

Penny and I waited in the lobby for another ten minutes or so, with her nursing all the while. The manager then approached and apologized, and I shared with them how difficult it is for women to nurse their babies because of harassment like that and that this kind of rudeness keeps many women from nursing at all. She defended the action by saying that some woman had complained, saying she hadn't wanted her children to see anyone nursing.

"That's the stupidest reason that can possibly be given," I said. "Children need to see babies nursing. Next time, you should inform the complainer that the nursing mother is doing the best thing possible for her baby and that if you don't want your children to see it, you can move to another place."

This second incident happened to my friend Lisa Goldstein. Her first baby, Moses, was a few weeks old when Lisa and her husband stopped at a small North Carolina café for breakfast. An older couple sat in a nearby booth, each having a cup of coffee. When Moses woke and got ready to start crying, Lisa unbuttoned her shirt to bring him to her left breast. Just then, she heard the man in the booth begin grumbling to his wife how disgusting this was. Almost without thinking, Lisa freed her right breast and turned slightly, just as her milk was letting down. A stream of milk arched from her breast through the air, landing dead center in the man's coffee cup. He immediately rose and stormed out of the café, followed by his wife, who turned to Lisa and her husband and gave them a triumphant thumbs-up. There is probably no nursing mother who has been harassed who wouldn't have loved to do that.

16

CREATING A BREASTFEEDING CULTURE

I sometimes wonder what nineteenth-century women's rights leaders such as Elizabeth Cady Stanton, Susan B. Anthony, and Sojourner Truth—had they been able to peek into the future—would have made of the lack of social and cultural assistance and acceptance that lactating mothers and their babies find in the United States today. The right of women to breastfeed their babies was not contested at all during their time—there was no other viable option. My guess is that it would have been hard for them to imagine that in less than a century after their deaths, mothers who chose to nurse their babies instead of feeding them manufactured formulas would meet with so many externally imposed obstacles.

The goals set by Stanton, Truth, and Anthony that were achieved during the twentieth-century long after their deaths were audacious. Because of these pioneers and the activists who followed them, women can now own property; divorce an abusive husband; vote; be elected to public office; be professors, executives, or astronauts; fly planes; and wear clothes that would have shocked everyone who lived in the nineteenth century (when women's ankles weren't supposed to be seen). All of these are solid and necessary gains, but today, even in states whose laws declare that breastfeeding cannot be considered "indecent exposure," the harassment of mothers for breastfeeding their babies when they leave their homes continues to a degree that is simply unacceptable. This rudeness to strangers and their babies can and must be stopped. In the nineteenth century, most U.S. mothers—if their health was good—nursed their babies, and people took it for granted that this elemental, nurturing act would have to take place as women traveled. I think it would have been hard for people in the nineteenth century to anticipate that advertising and marketing campaigns by infant-formula companies would become the dominant factor in parents' decisions about infant feeding and that infant-formula companies could so easily convince the medical profession to become the first promoters of their products.

With all of the problems women faced in the mid-nineteenth century, it wasn't necessary then to prove to the medical community and the general public that human milk was safe for human babies to drink. A century later, this was exactly what needed to happen. It was recognition of this necessity that led to the founding of La Leche League in the Chicago area in 1956. In large part, the influence of this organization prompted the research that persuaded the U.S. medical community that human milk is a safe food for human babies. Persuading the medical and nursing professions that it is a *superior* food is work that remains to us in the twenty-first century. Other essential work that must be done is the training of all health workers in how to care for women in ways that enhance, not undermine, their ability to breastfeed.

Stopping the promotion of artificial infant formulas in the United States (and the rest of the world) is just as necessary. Every one of the hospitals and birth centers in the United States in which babies are born should be Baby-Friendly—not a mere seventy-nine, nearly one-third of which are in California. We could be doing much better than this; several countries with far smaller populations than ours have many more Baby-Friendly hospitals per capita than we do. Consider the Philippines's 1,427; Brazil's 137; Thailand's 780, Mexico's 692, and tiny Ecuador's 141. Nigeria's 1,147, Iran's 376, Turkey's 83, Tunisia's 141, Malaysia's 144, and Egypt's 122, all have us beat. Norway, with one-sixtieth of our population, has thirty-five Baby-Friendly hospitals. Sweden, with approximately one-ninth of our population, has sixty-four. Forty-nine of Cuba's fifty-six hospitals are Baby-Friendly. Because these Baby-Friendly hospitals block the promotional schemes that the artificial-milk companies use to boost their profits, millions more babies now have a chance to be nourished on their mothers' milk than before the Baby-Friendly Hospital Initiative was launched. If we work hard and organize well enough to stop all kinds of advertising and promotion of these products in the United States, breastfeeding can become possible for millions more mothers here as well.

It's not that we haven't had our own activists and friends in the public-health community in the United States working diligently to increase rates of breastfeeding; it's that we have allowed a health-care industry responsible only to corporate boards of directors and stock-holders to take the place of what should be a health-care system designed for the benefit of all of our people. A profit-driven health-care industry has no reason to care about increasing breastfeeding rates (or doing anything else to promote health, for that matter), as doing so will do nothing to boost anyone's profits. I consider it a national embarrass-ment that our Department of Health and Human Services (DHHS) has never been able to collect solidly accurate statistics on breastfeeding rates for the first year of our babies' lives through any of its agencies. In fact, it is an infant-milk corporation whose data on breastfeeding rates, gathered in 1989 and again in 1995 by surveying a sample of mothers at hospital discharge and again at six months, are considered more dependable than any data-gathering our government services have ever attempted. There is something profoundly wrong with this.

The Department of Health and Human Services is given the power to set goals but not the power to achieve them. We have to change this.

What Can Happen When There Is No Accountability

Millions of Chinese parents found out the hard way in September 2008 that it's not a good idea to trust everything that comes in pretty pack-ages from corporations, with the government's seal of approval on them. That's when the news finally reached the public that more than twenty-two Chinese infant-formula companies had been selling prod-ucts adulterated with an industrial chemical called melamine, which can cause kidney stones or kidney failure. When blended into food, melamine (a crystalline white substance used in the manufacture of many plastics, fire retardants, and fertilizers) can make milk appear to have a higher protein content than it actually does; this helps watered-down milk pass quality tests in order to increase profits. At least six babies died, and another 300,000 were hospitalized with various manifestations of severe kidney disease. Anyone who has ever had a kidney stone knows how painful this disease is. Imagine having one when you're two months old. This is the same chemical that was implicated in the toxic-pet-food scandal of 2007 that killed thousands of people's pets all over the world.

Despite China's large number of Baby-Friendly hospitals (reportedly more than 6,000), artificial-milk products have been aggressively promoted as China races to catch up with the industrialized nations of the world—in everything profitable, that is, but not in regulation. Many rural women leave their babies in the care of the grandparents so they can work in the cities. Many others have pursued careers that make breastfeeding difficult or have had breast augmentation that interferes with their ability to breastfeed. Even farmers' wives who breastfed their babies during their first year of life have been convinced by aggressive advertising campaigns to wean earlier than their mothers would have and to introduce a formula-milk product as a staple. Many babies had been fed nothing but the poisoned milk formula from birth, with the result that babies a few months old had large kidney stones. A major reason for this public-health tragedy was that the Chinese government made the decision to stop product inspection for the twenty-two companies, since they had such exemplary records when they were still being regulated. Another big reason behind the public-health catastrophe is that China made the mistake of imitating U.S. health-industry fashions rather than following the lead of a country such as Norway, where women can have careers, be feminists, and still give their children the best start in life by breastfeeding them if possible.

Positive Steps Toward a Better Future

Believe it or not, Hollywood has begun to help the cause of promoting breastfeeding by making films that show women nursing their babies.

In real life, it has become fashionable for celebrities to be seen in public while pregnant and to let it be known they will breastfeed their babies. This is huge. We need tons more of this to make up for the devaluing of breastfeeding that has gone on for so many years. Women desperately need to see other women nursing their babies. Children everywhere should see babies being nurtured at their mother's breast. People who are afraid of allowing their children to know what breasts are for must clean up their minds.

We humans have to grow up and face the fact that our newborns' nervous systems are programmed in every way imaginable to be attracted to breasts. As newborns, it's what we most want to see, touch, smell, and taste. Even our sense of hearing leads us to the breast, since it is located so near our mother's beating heart, our place of security. Let's stop denying this, and we'll be moving in the direction of greater sanity.

How about a reality program on television that shows expert mothers (let the lactation consultants screen for the experts) nurturing their babies? Some of the mothers would be nursing their babies, and others (who perhaps weren't able to for some reason) would demonstrate how a baby should be held close to the breast while being bottle-fed. Surely Link TV could be persuaded to devote some airtime to this necessary educational service, provided that enough donations come in from viewers who request such programming. The kind of reality television that I'm talking about would not emphasize how to cover up properly while breastfeeding in public, as that would defeat the purpose of the show. We must see breasts and nipples wholesomely—not in a furtive way, but naturally.

Mother's milk is soul food for babies. The babies of the world need a lot more soul food.

ACKNOWLEDGMENTS

To the many people who helped me in the making of this book, I give my heartfelt thanks.

My grandmother Ina May Beard Stinson, who taught me to follow the example of women such as Elizabeth Cady Stanton, Susan B. Anthony, Helen Keller, and Jane Addams. They dreamed large, and she wanted me to know the challenges they overcame and how long it can take for change to come.

My parents, Ruth and Talford Middleton, who raised me to know that my body had the capacity to function perfectly—even if other people didn't think that possible. What a priceless gift that has been throughout my life!

My aunt Myra Middleton Savage, whose lessons about the needs of female mammals provided me with a firm grounding in nature's laws of birth and nurturing. These lessons proved invaluable when I began assisting women giving birth and nursing their babies.

My high school biology teacher, Leonard Cole, who taught me to keep an open mind, to question authority, and to look behind widely held assumptions that might later prove false.

My firstborn, Sydney Jane Kelley, for making my first breastfeeding experience easy and joyful—despite the hospital routines that kept us apart for most of her first five days of life.

My Malaysian (later Canadian) friend, Janice Ang, who in 1964 made me look at the negative effect that artificial milk feeding had on Chinese-Malaysian shopkeepers' babies and the irony that the more expensive form of infant feeding was far less healthy than breastfeeding would have been. She was the first person to open my eyes to the public health problems posed by the marketing of artificial milk substitutes in countries where safe substitutes are hard or impossible to ensure.

The women who gave birth on The Farm during the 1970s, who taught me how well women can breastfeed when newborns have the necessary access to their mothers just after birth.

Shunryu Suzuki Roshi, extraordinary teacher of Zen practice and author of *Zen Mind, Beginner's Mind,* who taught my husband, Stephen Gaskin, and by extension the people of The Farm community, that approaching problem solving with "beginner's mind" can be a good thing.

Stephen Gaskin, my husband, for attracting the people who followed the least sexist aspects of the counterculture of the 1960s to live in community with us. His support and patience throughout the writing of this book made my work on it as fun as it could possibly be.

The men who lived on The Farm from its beginnings to this day, who taught everyone in our community that even men who aren't used to public breastfeeding can accommodate to it and be healed in the process.

Eva, Samuel, and Paul, my children, for their love, their patience with my shortcomings as a parent, and the inspiration they have given me.

Asa Dotzler, who taught me how well newborns can crawl to the breast.

Margaret Nofziger and Louise Hagler, who taught me that some mothers have special needs and how to fill them.

Tisha Graham, whose generosity, breastfeeding expertise, and editorial skills helped me through difficult times during my writing process.

Eleanor Graf, lactation consultant, whose gentle words and teaching manner have transformed countless new mothers' breastfeeding problems into breastfeeding success.

Bonnie Reed, lactation consultant, whose reading of various parts of the manuscript and whose expertise about breast pumps was voluminous and helpful.

Gayla Groom, for her sympathetic ear and wise counsel when I struggled with the writing.

My midwives, for protecting me and my last three babies so beautifully during the magic time after their births.

Mary Kroeger, midwife, international maternal and child health consultant, whose untimely death from cervical cancer in 2004 followed the publication of her book *Impact of Birthing Practices on Breastfeeding* by only a few months. Ever the champion for women and babies whether she was working in any one of several African countries, Cambodia, Laos, Kazakhstan, Guatemala, Belize, or the United States, Mary made me promise to write this book: "Parents need the message as much as professionals do—that birth practices have a powerful impact on women's ability to breastfeed and that lactation knowledge is part of the essential body of knowledge that should be studied by all midwives, nurses, and physicians involved in birth and baby care."

Robyn Thompson, Aussie midwife and lactation consultant, whose generosity in inviting me along on several of her home lactation visits showed me how one-position-fits-all lactation advice given during short hospital stays can backfire on mothers who lack good follow-up lactation help such as that which she provides.

Suzanne Colson, research midwife, whose groundbreaking studies of lactation initiation have shown why mothers and babies need uninterrupted time with each other immediately after birth so they can do what should happen naturally.

Tina Greve, Norwegian midwife and lactation expert, who was always there to answer my questions about how Norway got so far ahead of North America when it comes to breastfeeding.

Juliana van Olphen-Fehr, midwife and midwifery educator, whose friendship, wisdom, and stories have nourished me at our every contact.

To Elizabeth and Ron Maxen, Jeanne and Leigh Kahan, David Frohman, Bernice Davidson, Kim Trainor, Angel Maharaj, Adanta Qubeck, Alison Blenkinsop, Alexandra Luzzatto, Allen Hagler, Anushka Bogoyevac, Bohdana Fasani, Catie Mehl, Andie Wyrick, Elizabeth Cochran, Janice Kahalley, Jenna Robertson, Jessica Coburn, Jennifer Moore, Julie Turner, Karen Strange, Natalie Carter, Kathryn Guernsey, Katie Riley, Kenda Burke, Neal Stiffelman, Virginia Gleser, Laura Hagler, Laura Lee, Laura Thompson, Leah Tarlen, Laureli Morrow, Linda J. Smith, Maddy Oden, Maja Vaskova, Mary Korduner, Nile Nash, Padraicin Ni Mhurchu, Pamela Hunt, Regi Kovaleski, Rosalie Kellman, Margaret

Wilmeth, Shannon Brinkman, Sherry Gaskin, Stacy Fine, Stefanie Rinza, Kenda Burke, Terry Barto, Tony Nenninger, Lorrie Leigh, Roberta Kachinsky, Leela Pratt, Árdis Kjartansdottir, Allison Gray, Leah Deragon, and all those who contributed ideas and stories.

To all those whom I may have unintentionally left off this list, please accept my thanks.

APPENDIX A: MEDICATIONS YOU MAY NEED

WHILE PREGNANT OR NURSING

Surveys in several countries have shown that ninety to ninety-nine percent of mothers will take some form of medication during the first postpartum week. Anecdotal evidence and surveys have shown that many women decide or are told not to breastfeed because of fear that medications they take might reach their babies through their milk. What these people don't know is that many medications that are transferred into mother's milk are destroyed in the baby's gut or are never absorbed into the baby's system. Unfortunately, though, a pediatrician who relies only on package inserts to evaluate possible negative effects of drugs on lactation may be unaware that these inserts usually contain statements designed more to provide legal protection for the pharmaceutical manufacturer than to protect babies who need their mothers' milk. The same goes for a pediatrician who uses the *Physicians' Desk Reference* (PDR) to evaluate drug safety, since this well-known reference is based upon manufacturers' package inserts—making it essentially worthless. If you live in Canada, your pediatrician is likely to refer to the *Compendium of Pharmaceuticals and Specialties* (CPS), which is essentially worthless with respect to breastfeeding information for the same reason.

Key Facts to Consider

- Most mothers can continue breastfeeding while taking a medication, without harming their babies. It's actually quite rare for women to have to completely stop nursing because of potential harm to their babies from a medication they must take.

- If a medication the mother needs is considered unsafe, there is usually another medication she could substitute that would pose no risk to her baby.

- Drug manufacturers have rarely funded studies of the effects of their drugs on breast milk, which explains the statements in package inserts that recommend cessation of breastfeeding.

- Amounts of medication reaching your baby through your milk on the first four to five days are extremely small because of the tiny amount of milk ingested during that time.

- The protective benefits of colostrum and milk during the first weeks of life almost always outweigh possible risks to babies posed by transfer of medications into your milk.

- It's best to avoid the newest medications on the market, as their effects are less likely to have been studied yet.

- Drugs with shorter half-lives are preferable to those with longer half-lives, such as some of the anticancer drugs.

- Herbal medications should also be used with caution, as some contain chemical substances that could be risky for your baby.

Our best authority on drugs and human milk is Dr. Thomas Hale's paperback book, *Medications and Mothers' Milk.* Dr. Hale, a clinical pharmacologist, recognizes the health benefits of breastfeeding for both mothers and babies and keeps his valuable book up to date by issuing new editions every few years. Many nursing mothers carry his book with them whenever they see a physician for their baby's or their own care. If your baby is born prematurely or ill, you might be wise to invest in a copy for yourself. Dr. Hale's book includes advice based upon published research regarding herbal medications that could affect your breastfed baby. Your lactation consultant almost certainly will own a copy.

Most medications that you might need to take at some point while nursing will result in only a tiny amount (around one percent) getting into your milk. Several factors are good to take into account in your decision-making. These include your medical needs, the age and maturity of your baby, the length of your treatment, the route of administration, whether or not the medication is absorbed by your baby's gut, and how much time passes after taking the medication before you nurse him. (Hint: If there is a drug that you must take during lactation, try to take your dose immediately after a feeding session, as this will minimize the amount of drug reaching your baby.)

Here are guidelines concerning the use of some commonly taken drugs:

Anti-allergy agents: People who are highly allergic to bee or wasp stings often carry epinephrine in case of a life-threatening allergic reaction. After epinephrine is given to a woman by injection, it is considered safe for her to continue nursing her baby.

Anti-allergy medications such as fexofenadine (Allegra) and diphenhydramine (Benadryl, Allerdryl, Insomnal, Nytol, Delixir, and Paedamin) are considered safe. There have been anecdotal reports of these medications suppressing milk production, but these haven't been substantiated. In general, though, a medication that produces a feeling of dryness in the nose and mouth may also have the effect of suppressing milk production.

Antibiotics: If, for any reason, it becomes necessary for you to take antibiotics during pregnancy, ask your midwife or doctor to make sure that any yeast infection that follows is resolved before you give birth. This precaution can prevent an oral thrush (yeast) infection from being transmitted to your baby during birth. Aviva Jill Romm's *The Natural Pregnancy Book* includes several good remedies, internal and external, for preventing and treating vaginal yeast infections. Sexual contact is another mode of transmission, so husbands need to be included in treatment as well as the mother and baby to break the cycle.

Most antibiotics that are commonly used are generally safe to take while breastfeeding. Small amounts do enter breast milk, and it is possible for some babies to show an allergic reaction, but most won't.

Ampicillin, amikacin, amoxicillin, gentamicin, methicillin, penicillin, tobramycin, and vancomycin (which is used for methicillin-resistant staph A, or MRSA, infections) are all considered safe for lactating mothers to take. Erythromycin and azithromycin are also considered safe, except when taken during the early postpartum period (when some newborns whose lactating mothers are taking erythromycin develop pyloric stenosis). Tetracyclines are considered safe, despite their bad reputation for causing discoloration and weakness of enamel of your child's second set of teeth. These effects happen only when a child is given large doses for more than three weeks. The same goes for doxycycline, a long half-life tetracycline antibiotic.

Furazolidone, a treatment for giardia lamblia, is considered safe in babies more than a month of age and is a good alternative to metronidazole (sometimes known as Flagyl, which is controversial: Some pharmacists advise mothers to stop nursing until twenty-four hours after the last dose, but guidelines in Canada's CPS state that discontinuing nursing while taking metronidazole is "overly conservative").

For most nursing mothers and babies, furazolidone and metronidazole pose no problem, and there is no need to stop nursing. If your baby is less than one month old and you are diagnosed with giardia, it would be advisable to wait.

Chinese herbalists use herbs such as garlic, licorice, pulsatilla (bai tou weng), scutellaria (huang qin), portulaca (ma chi xian), stemona (bai bu), and coptis (huang lian) for treating amoebic dysentery in pregnant and lactating mothers. All of these are considered safe within the tradition of Chinese herbal medicine; of these medications, Dr. Hale comments only on garlic, which he puts in his "moderately safe" risk category of medications that lack a foundation of published data regardless of how safe they may actually be.

Antidepressants and tranquilizers: These medications should be used with great caution. Some drugs in this category do produce noticeable effects in babies' behavior, particularly drowsiness. Many have not been on the market long enough for studies of their long-term effects to be carried out. For these reasons, counseling and lower-impact therapies are preferable, as long as they are effective. It's important to realize as well that too-sudden weaning can aggravate symptoms of depression because of shifts in hormone levels. Decisions about these medications should be made with a physician who has had experience working with breastfeeding mothers.

The herb St. John's wort, according to a study published recently by the *British Medical Journal,* is effective at suppressing anxiety and is virtually devoid of side effects.

Paroxetine (Paxil) is a much-prescribed serotonin reuptake inhibitor (SSRI). Very little of it gets into breast milk.

Sertraline (Zoloft) is another SSRI that is similar to Paxil and Prozac. Dr. Hale puts it in the category of medications for mother that pose only a remote risk for breastfed babies. Very small amounts of the drug get into breast milk.

Fluoxetine (Prozac, Apo-Fluoxetine, Novo-Fluoxetine, Lovan, and Zactin) is a third SSRI that is often prescribed for depression. Some side effects, such as fussiness, colic, and seizures, have been reported in babies of mothers taking these drugs. Dr. Hale remarks that he has received reports of several such cases himself, but he recommends that if a mother taking fluoxetine isn't able to tolerate a substitute medication, she should continue with the fluoxetine. (The reported problems were seen in babies less than six months old.)

Antifungals: Gentian violet and simple household remedies including vinegar or bicarbonate of soda compresses are good to try first in cases of overgrowth of thrush. Another remedy that many women swear by is grapefruit extract (one pill, or fifteen drops three times a day). If these don't do the job... clotrimazole and miconazole can be used topically for yeast infections, whether in a baby's mouth or for vaginal infections. Fluconazole is cleared for direct use in babies older than six months. The FDA has not given this clearance for babies younger than six months, but many pediatricians prescribe it anyway. Rarely, some negative effects to the liver have been reported, mostly in AIDS-infected babies taking other medications. Some of these babies had diarrhea, skin rashes, vomiting, and abdominal pain.

Antiparasitic medications: Avoid Lindane to treat scabies, as it stays in the body for a long time and is quite toxic. Permethrin is a better choice, and it can also be used in case of lice.

Mebendazole can be used for pinworms, roundworms, and hookworms, although it may inhibit milk production in some women.

Asthma medications: Asthma inhalers using ipratropium (DuoNeb) or albuterol (Proventil, Ventolin, Novo-Salmol, Asmavent, Respax, Respolin, Asmol, Salbulin, Salbuvent, and Salamol) are considered safe. Try not to swallow leftover medication after inhaler use.

Theophylline (aminophylline) may be used, but babies sometimes become jittery after its use.

Zafirlukast is considered safe.

Birth-control preparations: Avoid those products that contain estrogen, as they do inhibit milk production. The progestin-only pill (also called the mini-pill) is less likely to negatively affect lactation than those containing estrogen. If the progestin-only pill does reduce your milk supply, it would be good to switch to a hormone-free intrauterine device or barrier methods. Depo-Provera is somewhat controversial during nursing because of reports that it may cause lowered milk production, but these charges haven't been proven. Look in Resources for books on fertility awareness if you want to avoid any sort of medicated birth-control device.

Blood-pressure-control medications: These drugs haven't been well studied, since most women of breastfeeding age don't suffer from hypertension.

Esmolol and nisoldipine are considered safe.

Chemotherapy for cancer: Because of the toxicity of these drugs, it is better not to breastfeed.

Cold and cough medications: These drugs can be taken without prescription, but it's still advisable to use them cautiously while breastfeeding, as they can affect babies. For example, decongestants can cause babies to become irritable, and antihistamines can make them drowsy.

Be aware that medications containing pseudoephedrine may suppress milk supply.

Medications containing chlorpheniramine and phenylephrine may cause sedation in some babies.

Stay away from cough syrups containing codeine, such as Prometh VC with codeine cough syrup and promethazine HCL with codeine cough syrup. Another cold remedy to avoid is Rynatuss tablets (which contain chlorpheniramine and ephedrine).

In general, nasal sprays are safer for you to take than oral medications while breastfeeding. Such medications are best taken just after a feeding session to minimize the amount that is reaching the baby, and it's a good idea to limit their use to a day or two at a time. Using a saline nasal wash on a regular basis can prevent nasal, sinus, and ear problems caused by colds, allergies, infections, and exposure to pollution. See Resources.

Diuretics: These medications stimulate the kidneys to increase the amount of urine output. Sometimes they are prescribed to people with hypertension, but they are also sold as weight-loss drugs or antidotes for premenstrual fluid retention. They are best avoided during pregnancy and should be shunned during lactation (when you want more fluid, not less of it).

Migraine medications: Sumatriptan is considered safe. Little is known about other migraine medications.

Pain relievers: Avoid the use of fentanyl during labor, as it can inhibit milk production. The same goes for meperidine (Demerol or Pethidine), which makes the initiation of breastfeeding more difficult. Acetaminophen is considered the safest analgesic while breastfeeding. Narcotics (codeine, hydrocodone, and morphine) are generally safe but shouldn't be overused, as they may make the baby sleepy. According to the American Academy of Pediatrics (AAP), aspirin is generally safe if used with caution. However, continuous use could possibly cause bleeding in a breastfed baby. Low concentrations of aspirin do come into milk, and although no instances of Reye's syndrome or aspirin-related bleeding have been reported in breastfed babies, these side effects are considered possible, given sufficient exposure. For these reasons, acetaminophen or ibuprofen would be better choices. Pain relievers for dental work are safe. Nonsteroidal anti-inflammatory medications such as naproxen and piroxicam are considered safe if used for just a few days when a baby is more than a month of age.

Medications Not to Worry About While Breastfeeding

These include antacids, anticonvulsants, cortisone, insulin, laxatives, and thyroid medications. If you should need an MRI scan, you'll be given an injection of gadopentetate. Even though your radiologist may tell you to stop breastfeeding for twenty-four hours after this injection, only a tiny amount of this drug will get into your milk. The same goes for radiopaque iodine-containing agents. Continue nursing your baby.

Medications Not to Use While Breastfeeding

These include cancer chemotherapy drugs, radioactive drugs, long-term use of sedatives, pseudoephedrine (a decongestant), and ergot alkaloids such as migraine preps, ergotamine, and cabergoline (a relatively new drug used to treat pituitary tumors and other disorders you almost certainly don't have). Stay away from amphetamines, weight-loss products, and Parlodel (bromocriptine), a medication that was sometimes, and still is, prescribed to women who want to dry up their milk; several maternal deaths from stroke have occurred because of it.

Nonmedical Drugs

Alcohol: Alcohol does enter milk quickly after consumption, and large amounts taken over a short time can get your baby drunk. An occasional glass of wine or beer is not forbidden, but it's best to wait for an hour or two after a drink before you nurse. Drinking nearly every day is not a good idea, as heavy use may interfere with your ability to let down your milk.

Tobacco: Secondhand smoke is harmful to babies. If you are unable to stop smoking, do it outside to protect your baby.

Cocaine and heroin: Both of these drugs are highly addictive and should therefore be avoided.

Cannabis: Although this controversial herb is listed as contraindicated by the American Academy of Pediatrics, Dr. Hale puts it in a low-risk category, with the dose received being "insufficient to produce significant side effects in the infant."

Do You Have an Illness That Precludes Breastfeeding?

Women may find themselves diagnosed with illnesses during pregnancy that prompt questions regarding the safety of breastfeeding during the course of the illness or its treatment.

Cancer

The disease itself, in whatever part of the body it resides, is not contagious to others and is not transmitted via milk or bodily fluids. In general, the diagnostic tests that might be used when cancer is suspected need not interrupt breastfeeding. However, the use of radioactive compounds for diagnosis is incompatible with breastfeeding. If this is necessary, a mother should not continue breastfeeding for the duration of exposure and some time beyond (because it takes time for radioactivity to decline). If such a mother decides to express her milk to keep up her supply, her milk can be tested over time to determine its levels of radioactivity.

Chicken pox

Medical experts differ on whether women having chicken pox around the time of birth should be separated from their babies or not. (Some but not all babies get a severe case within the first ten days after birth if their mothers have chicken pox around the time of birth.) The period of contagion is about seven days. If the decision is for separation, milk should be expressed as often as possible and given to the baby. But the separation period in such a case can be shortened if the baby is given a varicella-zoster immune globulin injection, as these antibodies can prevent transmission and reduce the severity of infection.

Hepatitis A

Continue breastfeeding, but make sure that you wash your hands well with soap and water before handling your breasts or your baby's face, mouth, and hands.

Hepatitis B

If you have this form of hepatitis, the American Academy of Pediatrics Committee on Infectious Diseases recommends that your baby be given the hepatitis B immune globulin and hepatitis B virus vaccine soon after birth. Continue breastfeeding; this should be safe even before any immunization is given.

Hepatitis C

In general, research has not implicated breast milk as a transmitter for the hepatitis C virus, even though the milk may contain the virus. The reason for this may be that milk contains factors that prevent infectious agents from gaining entrance to the baby. Some pediatricians may advise against breastfeeding with cracked or bleeding nipples until the nipples are healed.

Herpes simplex I and II

Herpes simplex I (cold sores) and II (genital lesions) need not affect breastfeeding, as long as the baby does not touch the sores.

HIV (AIDS)

No conclusive evidence has been produced yet regarding which infant feeding method is preferable for the infants of HIV-positive mothers. In poor countries, many experts lean toward breastfeeding, given the many other dangers and challenges surrounding the use of artificial formulas. Many wealthy countries (where milk banks are available) discourage breastfeeding for HIV-positive mothers. In the end, each woman in this situation needs to come to her own best decision, with the help of her physician.

Human T-cell leukemia virus type 1

This type of virus is spread by sexual contact, sharing syringes, blood transfusions, and from mother to child during birth or breastfeeding. Those infected with the virus should not breastfeed, as such infection can cause leukemia and lymphoma.

Toxoplasmosis

This protozoal infection can be contracted through eating infected meat that is raw or undercooked or through contact with infected cat poop. Continue breastfeeding if you are being treated for it.

Tuberculosis

This infectious disease is compatible with breastfeeding, as long as it is considered safe for the mother to be with her baby. If temporary separation is necessary, milk should be expressed and discarded until the period of separation is over.

Herbs to Avoid While Breastfeeding

- Aloe
- Buckthorn bark and berry
- Cascara sagrada bark
- Coltsfoot leaf
- Extract of senna leaf, peppermint, and caraway oil
- Kava kava
- Indian snakeroot
- Rhubarb root
- Senna leaf
- Sage
- Uva ursi
- Jin bu huan
- Germander
- Mistletoe
- Skullcap

- Mate tea

- Pennyroyal oil

Breastfeeding is so good for your baby that there is almost never a good reason to stop doing it. Even if your baby gets some of a medication that has been prescribed for you, it would almost always be better for you to continue nursing than to start giving infant formula instead.

Appendix B: Recent Formula Recalls

June 2, 2008: Recall of about 13,000 cans of Abbott Laboratories' Calcilo XD Low-Calcium/Vitamin D-Free infant formula with iron powder in 14.1-oz. cans (400g). Reason: air contamination that causes spoilage of the food and foul smell.

May 28, 2007: Recall of Abbott's Ross Products' Similac Special Care 24cal./fl. oz. ready-to-feed premature infant formula with iron (5,000 cases). Reason: insufficient iron; using more than one month could result in anemia (not at all good for at-risk preemies).

December 14, 2006: The FDA told Nestlé that it might have to recall the group's Good Start Supreme infant formula with iron because tests showed it did not contain the minimum levels of calcium and phosphorus required under U.S. law. Nestlé disputed these findings, claiming that its tests were better than the FDA's. I could find no further information about how many cans of formula were involved, but none seem to have been recalled.

September 15, 2006: Recall of 200,000 bottles of Ross Products' Similac Advance with Iron liquid ready-to-feed formula (labeled to be used by

May 1, 2007) and 100,000 bottles of Similac Alimentum Advance (also for use by May 1, 2007). The FDA also had to warn that a lot of Similac Advance hospital-discharge gifts may have included some of the recalled products. Reason: not as much vitamin C as indicated on the label and dark, discolored liquid. Vitamin C deficiency could result from more than two to four weeks' use.

February 22, 2006: Recall of Mead Johnson's Gentlease powdered infant formula in 24-oz. cans (lot numbers BMJ19). Amount: 41,000 cans. Reason: metal splinters in cans. No one knows how many babies were fed formula with bits of metal before the manufacturer warned retailers to sell no more cans in that lot.

2005: Recall of Similac Advance with Iron formula powder. Almost 83,000 cans contained rigid polyvinyl chloride (PVC) particles and were distributed throughout the United States.

2005: Recall of Enfamil LactoFree with Lipil, 76,896 13-oz. concentrated-liquid cans. Reason: The formula had an "off odor, clumping, and product separation."

2003: Recall of Mead Johnson's EnfaCare Lipil, 12.9-oz. powdered formula for premature infants, 3,030 cans. Reason: contamination with *Enterobacter sakazakii*, which can cause sepsis, meningitis, and necrotizing enterocolitis, especially in premature or immunocompromised babies. In December 2002, 505 cases were shipped to hospitals, retail stores, and WIC clinics nationwide.

November 12, 2002: Recall of 1.5 million cans of Wyeth's powdered formula products. The tainted formula was sold under several names, including Baby Basics (Albertson's), Kozy Kids (Amway), CVS Soy Infant Formula, Hill Country Fare (HEB Grocery Stores), American Fare Little Ones (Kmart), HEB Baby Formula, HomeBest, Safeway Select, Healthy Best (Target), Walgreens, Parent's Choice (Walmart), Healthy Baby, and Perfect Choice. Reason: contamination with a food-borne pathogen that can cause blood infection, meningitis, or necrotizing enterocolitis (severe intestinal infection) in newborn infants.

2002: Recall of Portagen formula, 16-oz. powder; 17,358 cans were shipped nationwide in 2001 by Mead Johnson. Reason: A premature baby died in April 2001 from being given Portagen formula contaminated with *Enterobacter sakazakii.* Portagen is used for babies having trouble digesting fats.

2001: Recall of Carnation Follow-Up formula, 32-oz. liquid, 120 cans. Reason: excessive magnesium content, which can cause low blood pressure and irregular heartbeat. Walmart stores in nineteen Texas cities sold this stuff.

2001: Recall of Mead Johnson's LactoFree and Enfamil AR sample packs, distributed by physicians to their patients. Reason: Ingredients weren't listed on bottles. Babies allergic to milk protein ran the risk of serious or life-threatening allergic reaction if they drank this product.

2001: Recall of Mead Johnson's Nutramigen powder (3.7 million 16-oz. cans) and Nutramigen ready-to-feed (930,000 32-oz. cans). Reason: incorrect preparation directions in Spanish that could lead to seizures, irregular heartbeat, or death if the formula was used over several days. Babies who were already ill or who lived in hot climates were at greater risk for potentially fatal complications. The formula was distributed nationwide, as well as in Guam, the Dominican Republic, and Puerto Rico. According to lactation consultant Marsha Walker, the product was allowed to remain in stores, with parents being expected to notice the correct preparation instructions in Spanish as tear-off sheets.

2000: Recall of repackaged infant formula: Isomil powder and concentrate; Similac with iron, low-iron powder, and concentrate; Neosure powder; Enfamil low-iron and with-iron powder; Enfamil LactoFree powder; Prosobee soy powder. Reason: misbranded packaging.

2000: Recall of Nestlé Carnation Good Start, Alsoy, and Follow-Up in 13-oz. concentrate (2.5 million cans). Reason: processing screwup, with temperatures not high enough to ensure sterility. Maybe not such a good start after all.

On March 12, 2008, Reuters news agency reported that Nestlé, the world's largest food company, was recalling a batch of infant formula that had been contaminated with excessive levels of copper, iron, and zinc, causing an unknown number of babies to suffer from vomiting and diarrhea. The Swiss parent company told Reuters that the recalled cans of formula were so foul-smelling that no baby would have swallowed them. Nevertheless, at least fifteen customer complaints followed the news report in certain African countries, so some babies did swallow the stuff. There have been no reports of Nestlé and the other artificial-milk companies paying restitution for the illnesses their products have caused.

Are you surprised by the length of this list? Were any of these recalls publicized well enough for you to have heard about them? I won't be surprised if your answer is no. FDA's website does not archive recall information. This means that FDA's recall notices are posted for only a few weeks before being removed. How many U.S. babies have been made sick or died from drinking some of the "recalled" products mentioned above is unknown, because we currently have no reliable way of gathering this information.

China's Melamine Scandal and Some Lessons to Be Learned from It

Following the first official revelations in September 2008, of the melamine-tainted infant-formula scandal in China that killed at least six babies, put another 300,000 in the hospital and permanently damaged the kidneys of an unknown number of those who were hospitalized, the FDA was quick to reassure the U.S. public that there was nothing to fear about contaminated formula in the United States. Dr. Stephen Sundlof, director of the FDA's Center for Food Safety and Applied Nutrition, told reporters on October 3, 2008, that none of the five manufacturers that supply infant formula to the United States uses any milk or milk products from China.[1]

Sundlof went on to say that the FDA had determined that for all foods *except infant formula,* only those with amounts of melamine less than

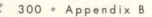

2.5 parts per million were acceptable. As for levels in infant formula, the Associated Press quoted Sundlof: "FDA is currently unable to establish any level of melamine and melamine-related compounds in infant formula that does not raise public health concerns." This statement was widely taken to mean there was a policy of zero tolerance of melamine in U.S. infant formula. According to a statement by the Grocery Manufacturers Association to its members: "FDA could not identify a safe level for melamine and related compounds in infant formula; thus it can be concluded they will not accept any detectable melamine in infant formula."[2]

Less than two months later, the FDA reported that it had found trace amounts of melamine in the U.S. formulas produced by the big three companies: Nestlé, Mead Johnson, and Abbott (their infant formula constitutes ninety percent of that sold in the United States). At the same time, the agency stated a new standard for melamine in baby formula that would consider products with less than 1 part per million of melamine acceptable, provided that cyanuric acid (a melamine byproduct) was not also present.

Consumers Union called the FDA decision "seriously flawed" and medically risky because parents may feed their babies more than one product. Author James E. McWilliams, in an article for Slate.com, called the FDA decision "the arbitrary adjustment of allowable levels of a contaminant."[3] According to Urvashi Rangan, a senior scientist with the Consumers Union, "The FDA needs to step up and expand melamine testing. The failure to properly inform people about these findings undermines consumer confidence in a fundamental product that millions of parents depend on."[4]

Remarkably, the new U.S. standard for melamine allows for twenty times as much of the chemical in infant formula as Taiwan's standard of 0.5 part per million. Why is this standard not possible in the United States?

APPENDIX C: THE TEN STEPS
TO SUCCESSFUL BREASTFEEDING

A Joint WHO/UNICEF Statement, Geneva, Switzerland, 1989

Every facility or agency providing maternity services and care of newborn infants should:

- Have a written breastfeeding policy that is routinely communicated to all health-care staff.

- Train all health-care staff in skills necessary to implement this policy.

- Inform all pregnant women about the benefits and management of breastfeeding.

- Help mothers initiate breastfeeding within one half-hour of birth.

- Show mothers how to breastfeed and maintain lactation, even if they should be separated from their infants.

- Give newborn infants no food or drink other than breast milk, unless medically indicated.

- Practice rooming-in—that is, allow mothers and infants to remain together twenty-four hours a day.

- Encourage breastfeeding on demand.

- Give no artificial teats or pacifiers (also called dummies or soothers) to breastfeeding infants.

- Foster the establishment of breastfeeding support groups and refer mothers to them on discharge from the hospital or clinic.

Resources

Organizations

Adoptive Breastfeeding Resource
www.fourfriends.com/abrw/

African-American Breastfeeding Alliance (AABA)
877-677-1691
www.aabaonline.com

Breastfeeding After Reduction
www.bfar.org

International Lactation Consultant Association (ILCA)
919-861-5577
www.ilca.org

La Leche League International
847-519-7730
Breastfeeding Helpline: 800-LALECHE (525-3243)
www.llli.org

National Women's Health Information Center
Breastfeeding Helpline: 800-994-9662
www.4woman.gov/breastfeeding

Activist Mothers

Holistic Moms Network
877-HOL-MOMS (465-6667)
www.holisticmoms.org

International Moms Clubs
www.momsclub.org

Lactnet
www.lsoft.com/scripts/wl.exe?SL1=LACTNET&H=COMMUNITY.
LSOFT.COM

League of Maternal Justice
www.leagueofmaternaljustice.com

Mocha Moms, Inc.
www.mochamoms.org

MomsRising
www.momsrising.org

Motherhood Project
www.motherhoodproject.org

Mothers International Lactation Campaign (MILC)
www.womantowomancbe.wordpress.com

Mothers & More
630-941-3553
www.mothersandmore.org

Mothers Movement Online (MMO)
www.mothersmovement.org

Mothers Ought to Have Equal Rights
www.mothersoughttohaveequalrights.org

National Association of Mothers' Centers (NAMC)
877-939-MOMS (939-6667)
www.motherscenter.org

SearchMothers
www.searchmothers.com

Books

Medications and Mothers' Milk, 12th Edition
Dr. Thomas Hale
Pharmasoft Publishing, 2008
http://neonatal.ama.ttuhsc.edu/lact/ is Dr. Hale's informative website.
Look to it for updates on new medications.
www.ibreastfeeding.com

Mothering Multiples: Breastfeeding & Caring for Twins or More!
Karen Kerkhoff Gromada

Defining Your Own Success: Breastfeeding After Breast Reduction Surgery
Diana West
www.bfar.org

The Natural Pregnancy Book
Aviva Jill Romm

The Breastfeeding Café
Barbara Behrmann

The Milk Memos: How Real Moms Learned to Mix Business with Babies—and How You Can, Too
Cate Colburn-Smith and Andrea Serrette

Clinics in Human Lactation: Non-Pharmacologic Treatments for Depression in New Mothers: Evidence-Based Support of Omega-3s, Bright Light Therapy, Exercise, Social Support, Psychotherapy, and St. John's Wort
Kathleen Kendall-Tackett, PhD, IBCLC

Clinics in Human Lactation: Breastfeeding the Late-Preterm Infant: Improving Care and Outcomes
Marsha Walker, RN, IBCLC

Impact of Birthing Practices on Breastfeeding: Protecting the Mother and Baby Continuum
Mary Kroeger with Linda J. Smith

The Ultimate Breastfeeding Book of Answers: The Most Comprehensive Problem-Solving Guide to Breastfeeding from the Foremost Expert in North America, Revised & Updated Edition
Jack Newman, MD, and Teresa Pitman
www.drjacknewman.com is Dr. Newman's informative website.

Fit to Bust
Alison Blenkinsop
Visit Alison's website at www.linkable.biz.

The Happiest Baby on the Block (book and DVD)
Harvey Karp, MD
www.thehappiestbaby.com

Helpful Handouts

The Diaper Diary (for knowing what color and how much poo to expect) and Pumping Milk for Your Premature Baby
www.lactnews.com/ddiary.html

L. Stokowski. Newborn jaundice. *Advances in Neonatal Care* 2002; 2:115.

Contemporary Pediatrics. Guide for parents going home with your late-preterm infant.
www.modernmedicine.com/Parent+Guides/Parent-Guide-Going
-home-with-your-late-preterm-inf/ArticleStandard/Article/detail/
473739?contextCategoryId=6465

Late-Preterm (Near-Term) Infant: What Parents Need to Know
www.awhonn.org/awhonn/content.do?name=02_PracticeResources/
2C3_Focus_NearTermInfant.htm

Films

Orgasmic Birth
www.orgasmicbirth.com

The Business of Being Born
www.businessofbeingborn.com

The Story of the Weeping Camel
This Mongolian documentary depicts a mother camel with post-traumatic stress, who refuses to nurse her calf. A ritual involving music solves the problem.
www.nationalgeographic.com/weepingcamel/

Breast is Best
www.inamay.com

Pregnant in America: A Nation's Miscarriage
www.pregnantinamerica.com

Dr. Jack Newman's Visual Guide to Breastfeeding
Available in English, French, and with Spanish subtitles

Being an Active Patient

For Carol Melcher's Intervention for Newborns, Google "Breastfeeding Hospital Policy Recommendation Policy #5"
This "intervention" has been described as a new "approach to training resistant hospital staff."

Supplies You May Need

Breast Pumps:
Medela, Inc.'s Breastfeeding National Network at 800-TELLYOU (835-5968) or www.medela.com

Ameda Egnell at 800-323-4060
www.ameda.com

Foley Cup:
Go to www.foleycup.com or email info@foleycup.com or phone 888–463–2688 for ordering information

Pillows:
For Twins: EZ-2-Nurse Twins pillow or the NurseMate pillow

Vitamin B12 for Vegans or Vegetarians:
Good-Tasting Nutritional Yeast
www.healthy-eating.com

The Miracle Blanket:
www.MiracleBlanket.com

Dr. Hana's Nasal Cleansing System
www.nasopure.com

Services for Sick Babies

International Chiropractic Pediatric Association
610-565-2360
www.icpa4kids.com

Tetralogy Service
www.otispregnancy.org

The Craniosacral Therapy Association of North America
www.craniosacraltherapy.org

Fertility Awareness

Taking Charge of Your Fertility: The Definitive Guide to Natural Birth Control, Pregnancy Achievement, and Reproductive Health, Revised Edition
Toni Weschler

Signs of Fertility: The Personal Science of Natural Birth Control
Margaret Nofziger

Honoring Our Cycles: A Natural Family Planning Workbook
Katie Singer

Your Fertility Signals: Using Them to Achieve or Avoid Pregnancy Naturally
Merryl Winstein

Notes

Notes for Introduction

1. American Academy of Pediatrics, Policy Statement. Breastfeeding and the Use of Human Milk. *Pediatrics.* 2005; 115:496–506.

2. Heinig, M.J. Host defense benefits of breastfeeding for the infant: effect of breastfeeding duration and exclusivity. *Pediatric Clinics of North America.* 2001; 48:106–123, ix.

3. Cochi, S.L., D.W. Fleming, et al. Risk factors for primary invasive Haemophilus influenzae disease increased risk from day care attendance and school-aged household members. *Journal of Pediatrics.* 1986; 108(6): 887–896.

4. Takala, A.K., J. Eskola, et al. Risk factors of invasive Haemophilus influenzae type b disease among children in Finland. *Journal of Pediatrics.* 1989; 115:694–701.

5. Kramer, M.S., T. Guo, et al. Infant growth and health outcomes associated with 3 compared with 6 months of exclusive breastfeeding. *American Journal of Clinical Nutrition.* 2003; 78:291–295.

6. Blaymore, B.J., A. Ferguson, et al. Human milk reduces outpatient upper respiratory symptoms in premature infants during their first year of life. *Journal of Perinatology.* 2002; 22:354–359.

7. Dewey, K.G., M.J. Heinig, et al. Differences in morbidity between breast-fed and formula-fed infants. *Journal of Pediatrics.* 1995; 126:696–702.

8. Lopez-Alarcón, M., S. Villalpando, et al. Breast-feeding lowers the frequency and duration of acute respiratory infection and diarrhea in infants under six months of age. *Journal of Nutrition.* 1997; 127:436–443.

9. Schanler, R.J., R.J. Shulman, et al. Feeding strategies for premature infants: beneficial outcomes of feeding fortified human milk versus preterm formula. *Pediatrics.* 1999; 103:1150–1157.

10. Lucas, A., and T.J. Cole. Breast milk and neonatal necrotising enterocolitis. *Lancet.* 1990; 336:1519–1523.

11. Saarinen, U.M. Prolonged breastfeeding as prophylaxis for recurrent otitis media. *Acta Paediatrica Scandinavica.* 1982; 71:567–571.

12. Marild, S., S. Hansson, et al. Protective effect of breastfeeding against urinary tract infection. *Acta Paediatrica Scandinavica.* 2004; 93:164–168.

13. Hylander, M.A., D.M. Strobino, et al. Human milk feedings and infection among very low birth weight infants. *Pediatrics.* 1998; 102(3). Available at: www.pediatrics.org/cgi/content/full/102/3/e38.

14. Hylander, M.A., D.M. Strobino, et al. Association of human milk feedings with a reduction in retinopathy of prematurity among very low birthweight infants. *Journal of Perinatology.* 2001; 21:356–362.

15. Chen, A., and W.J. Rogan. Breastfeeding and the risk of postneonatal death in the United States. *Pediatrics.* 2004; 113(5). Available at: www.pediatrics.org/cgi/content/full/113/5/e435.

16. Cunningham, A.S., D.B. Jelliffe, et al. Breast-feeding and health in the 1980s: a global epidemiological review. *The Journal of Pediatrics.* 1991; 68.

17. McVea, K.L., P.D. Turner, et al. The role of breastfeeding in sudden infant death syndrome. *Journal of Human Lactation.* 2000; 16:13–20.

18. Pettit, D.J., M.R. Forman, et al. Breastfeeding and the incidence of non-insulin-dependent diabetes mellitus in Pima Indians. *Lancet.* 1997; 350:166–168.

19. Bener, A., S. Denic, et al. Longer breastfeeding and protection against childhood leukemia and lymphomas. *European Journal of Cancer.* 2001; 37:234–238.

20. Armstrong, J., and J.J. Reilly, Child Health Information Team. Breastfeeding and lowering the risk of childhood obesity. *Lancet.* 2002; 359:2003–2004.

21. Owen, C.G., P.H. Whincup, et al. Infant feeding and blood cholesterol: a study in adolescents and a systematic review. *Pediatrics.* 2002; 110:597–608.

22. Chulada, P.C., S.J. Arbes Jr., et al. Breast-feeding and the prevalence of asthma and wheeze in children: analyses from the Third National Health and Nutrition Examination Survey, 1988–1994. *Journal of Allergy and Clinical Immunology.* 2003; 111:328–336.

23. Lucas, A., R. Morley, et al. Randomised trial of early diet in preterm babies and later intelligence quotient. *British Medical Journal.* 1998; 317:1481–1487.

24. Mortensen, E.L., K.F. Michaelsen, et al. The association between duration of breastfeeding and adult intelligence. *Journal of the American Medical Association.* 2002; 287:2365–2371.

25. Horwood, L.J., and D.M. Fergusson. Breastfeeding and later cognitive and academic outcomes. *Pediatrics.* 1998; 101(1). Available at: www.pediatrics.org/cgi/content/full/101/1/e9.

26. Gray, L., L.W. Miller, et al. Breastfeeding is analgesic in healthy newborns. *Pediatrics.* 2002; 109:590–593.

27. Carbajal, R., S. Veerapen, et al. Analgesic effect of breast feeding in term neonates: randomised controlled trial. *British Medical Journal.* 2003; 326:13.

28. Chua, S., S. Arulkumaran, et al. Influence of breastfeeding and nipple stimulation on postpartum uterine activity. *British Journal of Obstetrics & Gynaecology.* 1994; 101:804–805.

29. Cooney, K., et al. An assessment of the nine-month Lactational Amenorrhea Method (MAMA-9) in Rwanda. *Studies in Family Planning.* 1996; 27(3):162–171.

30. Kennedy, K.I., M.H. Labbok, et al. Lactational amenorrhea method for family planning. *International Journal of Gynaecology & Obstetrics.* 1996; 54:55–57.

31. Diaz, S., et al. Contraceptive efficacy of lactational amenorrhea in urban Chilean women. *Contraception.* 1991; 43(4):335–352.

32. Dewey, K.G., M.J. Heinig, et al. Maternal weight-loss patterns during prolonged lactation. *American Journal of Clinical Nutrition.* 1993: 58:162–166.

33. Collaborative Group on Hormonal Factors in Breast Cancer. Breast cancer and breastfeeding: collaborative reanalysis of individual data from 47 epidemiological studies in 30 countries, including 50,302 women with breast cancer and 96,973 women without the disease. *Lancet.* 2002; 360:187–195.

34. Lee, S.Y., M.T. Kim, et al. Effect of lifetime lactation on breast cancer risk: a Korean women's cohort study. *International Journal of Cancer.* 2003; 105:390–393.

35. Tryggvadottir, L., H. Tulinius, et al. Breastfeeding and reduced risk of breast cancer in an Icelandic cohort study. *American Journal of Epidemiology.* 2001; 154:37–42.

36. Jernstrom, H., J. Lubinski, et al. Breast-feeding and the risk of breast cancer in BRCA1 and BRCA2 mutation carriers. *Journal of the National Cancer Institute.* 2004; 96:1094–1098.

37. Ing, R., J.H.C. Ho, et al. Unilateral breast-feeding and breast cancer. *Lancet.* 1977; 2:124–127.

38. Rosenblatt, K.A., and D.B. Rhomas. Lactation and the risk of epithelial ovarian cancer. WHO Collaborative Study of Neoplasia

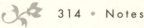

and Steroid Contraceptives. *International Journal of Epidemiology.* 1993; 22:192–197.

39. Cumming, R.G., and R.J. Klineberg. Breastfeeding and other reproductive factors and the risk of hip fractures in elderly women. *International Journal of Epidemiology.* 1993; 22:684–691.

40. Lopez, J.M., G. Gonzalez, et al. Bone turnover and density in healthy women during breastfeeding and after weaning. *Osteoporosis International.* 1996; 6:153–159.

41. Paton, L.M., J.L. Alexander, et al. Pregnancy and lactation have no long-term deleterious effect on measures of bone mineral in healthy women: a twin study. *American Journal of Clinical Nutrition.* 2003; 77:707–714.

Notes for Chapter 1

1. Uvnäs Moberg, Kerstin. *The Oxytocin Factor: Tapping the Hormone of Calm, Love, and Healing.* Cambridge, Mass.: Da Capo Press, 2003.

2. Ibid.

3. Odent, M. *Birth and Breastfeeding.* East Sussex, England: Clairview Books, 2003.

4. Lawrence, R.A. *Breastfeeding: A Guide for the Medical Profession: Sixth Edition.* St. Louis: C. V. Mosby, 2005.

5. Roberts, R.L., et al. Prolactin levels are elevated after infant carrying in parentally inexperienced common marmosets. *Physiology and Behavior.* 2001; 72(5):713–720.

6. Fleming, A.S., et al. Testosterone and prolactin are associated with emotional responses to infant cries in new fathers. *Hormones and Behavior.* 2002; 42(4):399–413.

7. Lawrence, R.A., op. cit.

8. Cregan, M., and P. Hartmann. Computerized breast measurement from conception to weaning: clinical implications. *Journal of Human Lactation.* 1999; 15(2):89–96.

Notes for Chapter 2

1. Hurst, N. Lactation after augmentation mammoplasty. *Obstetrics & Gynecology.* 1996; 87(1):30–34.

2. Levine, J., and N. Ilowite. Sclerodermalike esophageal disease in children breast-fed by mothers with silicone breast implants. *Journal of the American Medical Association.* 1994; 271:213–216.

3. Grigg, M., et al, Editors, Institute of Medicine. *Information for Women about the Safety of Silicone Breast Implants.* Washington, D.C.: National Academy Press, 2000.

4. Kjoller, K., et al. Health outcomes in offspring of mothers with breast implants. *Pediatrics.* 1998; 102(5):1112–1115.

5. Kjoller, K., et al. Health outcomes in offspring of Danish mothers with cosmetic breast implants. *Annals of Plastic Surgery.* 2002; 48(3):238–245.

6. Institute of Medicine. Dietary reference intakes: calcium, phosphorus, magnesium, vitamin D, and fluoride. Washington, D.C.: National Academy Press, 1997.

7. Prentice, A. Calcium requirements of breast-feeding mothers. *Nutrition Reviews.* 1998; 56(4):124–130.

Notes for Chapter 3

1. Sosa, R., J. Kennell, M. Klaus, et al. The effect of a supportive companion on perinatal problems, length of labor, and mother–infant interaction. *New England Journal of Medicine.* 1980; 303:597–600.

2. Klaus, M., J. Kennell, S.S. Robertson, et al. Effects of social support during parturition on maternal and infant morbidity. *British Medical Journal.* 1986; 293(6547):585–587.

3. Kennell, J., M. Klaus, et al. Continuous emotional support during labor in a U.S. hospital. *Journal of the American Medical Association.* 1991; 265(17):2197–2201.

4. Simkin, P. *The Birth Partner: Everything You Need to Know to*

Help a Woman Through Childbirth. Third Edition. Boston: Harvard Common Press, 2007.

5. Caldeyro-Barcia, R. The influence of maternal position during second stage of labor. *Birth and Family Journal*. 1979; 6(1):31–42.

6. Poor, M., and J.C. Foster. Epidural and no epidural anesthesia: Differences between mothers and their experience of birth. *Birth*. 1985; 12:205–212.

7. Lieberman, E., K. Davidson, et al. Changes in fetal position during labor and their association with epidural anesthesia. *Obstetrics & Gynecology*. 2005; 105(5 Pt 1):974–982.

8. Baumgarder, D.J., P. Muehl, et al. Effect of labor epidural anesthesia on breast-feeding of healthy full-term newborns delivered vaginally. *Journal of the American Board of Family Practice*. 2003; 16:7–13.

9. Leighton, B., and S. Halpern. The effects of epidural anesthesia on labor, maternal and neonatal outcomes. *American Journal of Obstetrics & Gynecology*. 2002; 186:569–577.

10. Halpern, S.H., T. Levine, et al. Effect of labor analgesia on breast-feeding success. *Birth*. 1999; 26(2):83–88.

11. Belsey, E.M., D.B. Rosenblatt, et al. The influence of maternal analgesia on neonatal behaviour: pethidine. *British Journal of Obstetrics & Gynaecology*. 1981; 88:398–406.

12. Belfrage, P., L.O. Boreus, et al. Neonatal depression after obstetrical analgesia with pethidine. The role of injection-delivery time interval and the plasma concentrations of pethidine and norpethidine. *Acta Obstetricia et Gynecologica Scandinavica*. 1981; 60:43–49.

13. Righard, L., and M.O. Alade. Effect of delivery room routines on success of first breast-feed. *Lancet*. 1990; 336:1105–1107.

14. Crowell, M.K., P.D. Hill, et al. Relationship between obstetric analgesia and time of effective feeding. *Journal of Nurse Midwifery*. 1994; 39(3):150–156.

15. Mercer, J., B. Vohr, et al. Delayed cord clamping in very preterm infants reduces the incidence of intraventricular hemorrhage and late-onset sepsis: a randomized, controlled trial. *Pediatrics*. 2006; 117:1235–1242.

16. Christensson, K., C. Siles, et al. Temperature, metabolic adaptation and crying in healthy full-term newborns cared for skin-to-skin or in a cot. *Acta Paediatrica*. 1992; 81:488–493.

17. Righard, L., and M.O. Alade, op. cit.

18. Varendi, H., R.H. Porter, et al. Does the newborn find the nipple by smell? *Lancet*. 1994; 344(8928):989–990.

19. Varendi, H., and R.H. Porter. Breast odour as the only maternal stimulus elicits crawling toward the odour source. *Acta Paediatrica*. 2001; 90(4):372–375.

20. Ferber, S.G., and R. Makhoul. The effect of skin-to-skin contact (kangaroo care) shortly after birth on the neurobehavioral responses of the term newborn: a randomized, controlled trial. *Pediatrics*. 2004; 113(4):858–865.

21. Wagner, M., with S. Gunning. *Creating Your Birth Plan: The Definitive Guide to a Safe and Empowering Birth*. New York: The Berkeley Publishing Group, Penguin Group (USA) Inc., 2006.

22. Righard, L., and K. Frantz. *Delivery Self Attachment* (video). Sunland, Calif.: Geddes Productions, 1992.

23. Levin, A. The Mother-Infant Unit at Tallinn Children's Hospital, Estonia: A Truly Baby-Friendly Unit. *Birth*. 1994; 21(1):39–44.

24. Svensson, K., A. Matthiesen, et al. Night rooming-in: Who decides? An example of staff influence on mother's attitude. *Birth*. 2005; 32(2):99–106.

25. Quoted in editorial by Diony Young. *Birth*. 2005; 32(3):161–163.

26. Baby-Friendly USA. Website: www.babyfriendlyusa.org.

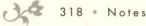

27. Alvarez, L. Norway leads industrial nations back to breast-feeding. *New York Times.* October 21, 2003.

28. Harris, G. More mothers breast-feed, in first months at least. *New York Times.* May 1, 2008.

29. Young, Diony. *Birth* 2005. 32(3): 161–163.

30. Ibid.

Notes for Chapter 4

1. Colson, S.D., J.H. Meek, et al. Optimal positions for the release of primitive neonatal reflexes stimulating breastfeeding. *Early Human Development.* 2008; 84:441–449.

2. Colson, S.D. Biological suckling facilitates exclusive breastfeeding from birth, a pilot study of 12 vulnerable infants. Dissertation submitted as course requirement of MSc in Midwifery Studies. London: South Bank University, June 2000.

3. Colson, S., L. DeRooy, and J. Hawdon. Biological nurturing increases duration of breastfeeding for a vulnerable cohort. *MIDIRS Midwifery Digest.* 2003; 13(1):92–97.

Notes for Chapter 5

1. Lawrence, R. *Breastfeeding: A Guide for the Medical Profession: Fifth Edition.* St. Louis: C.V. Mosby, 1999; p. 398.

Notes for Chapter 7

1. Fitzpatrick, M.G. SIDS and The Toxic Gas Theory (letter). *New Zealand Medical Journal.* October 9, 1998.

2. Kapuste, H. *Giftige Gase im Kinderbett* (Toxic Gases in Infants' Beds). *Zeitschrift fuer Umweltmedizin.* January–April 2002; No. 44: 18–20.

1. Jones, K.G., and R. Matheny. Relationship between infant feeding and exclusion rate from child care because of illness. *Journal of the American Dietetic Association.* 1993; 93(7):8098–9011.

2. Workplace Breastfeeding Support, United States Breastfeeding Committee. 2002; www.usbreastfeeding.org/Issue-Papers/Workplace.pdf.

3. Talayero, J.M.P., M. Lizán-Garcia, et al. Full breastfeeding and hospitalization as a result of infections in the first year of life. *Pediatrics.* 2006; 118:92–99.

4. Workplace Breastfeeding Support, United States Breastfeeding Committee. 2002; www.usbreastfeeding.org/Issue-Papers/Workplace.pdf.

5. Bailey, D. Breastfeeding: the best investment. Raleigh, N.C.: International Lactation Consultant Association, 1998; www.wicworks.ca.gov/breastfeeding/EmployerResources/bf_bestinvestment.pdf. The Business Case for Breastfeeding. http://ask.hrsa.gov/detail.cfm?PubID=MCH00249+recommended=1.

6. Centers for Disease Control and Prevention. Third National Report on Human Exposure to Environmental Chemicals. Atlanta, Ga.: CDC, 2005; www.cdc.gov/exposurereport/report.htm.

7. Rust, Susanne, and Meg Kissinger. Tests find BPA in "safe" food containers. *Milwaukee Journal Sentinel.* November 17, 2008.

8. Institute for Agriculture and Trade Policy (www.iatp.org/foodandhealth) is a good website for learning which products are toxic and which are not.

Notes for Chapter 14

1. Lee-St. John, J. Outsourcing breast milk. *Time.* April 19, 2007.

2. Jameson, M. Feeding a need. *Los Angeles Times,* April 11, 2005.

3. Baumgardner, J. Breast friends. www.babble.com. January 22, 2007.

4. Lee-St. John, J., op. cit.

5. Palmer, G. *The Politics of Breastfeeding.* London: Pandora, 1988.

6. Wieschhoff, H. *Bulletin of the History of Medicine.* December 1940; 7(10): 1403–1415.

7. Fildes, V. *Breasts, Bottles, & Babies: A History of Infant Feeding.* Edinburgh: Edinburgh University Press, 1986.

Notes for Appendix B

1. Reinberg, Steve. FDA rules how much melamine is too much. *U.S. News & World Report* (Usnews.com), October 3, 2008.

2. Lowy, Joan, and Justin Pritchard. FDA sets melamine standard for baby formula. The Associated Press, www.abcnews, November 29, 2008.

3. McWilliams, James E. Tainted government: How did the Food and Drug Administration let melamine into the U.S. food supply? Slate.com, December 29, 2008.

4. Press Release: With new FDA infant formula test data, CU urges expanded testing, recalls. January 9, 2009, www.consumersunion.org.

IMAGE CREDITS AND PERMISSIONS

Image #1, page 19, David Frohman
Image #2, page 22, Sukree Sukplang/Reuters
Image #3, page 24, Luis Gonzalez
Image #4, page 36, Ina May Gaskin
Image #5, page 37, Ina May Gaskin
Image #6, page 38, Ina May Gaskin
Image #7, page 39, Kim Trainor
Image #8, page 42, Ina May Gaskin
Image #9, page 61, Massimo Listri/CORBIS
Image #10, page 72, Ina May Gaskin
Image #11, page 82, David Frohman
Image #12, page 83, Luis Gonzalez
Image #13, page 85, Luis Gonzalez
Image #14, page 87, Ina May Gaskin
Image #15, page 90, Ina May Gaskin
Image #16, page 92, Ina May Gaskin
Image #17, page 94, Leah Deragon
Image #18, page 96, Ina May Gaskin
Image #19, page 98, Ina May Gaskin

Image #20, page 109, David Frohman

Image #21, page 110, Kim Trainor

Image #22, page 117, Ina May Gaskin

Image #23, page 138, Bernice Davidson

Image #24, page 160, Ina May Gaskin

Image #25, page 203, Kim Trainor

Image #26, page 232, Photograph taken from the Internet; source
untraceable

Image #27, page 254, Ina May Gaskin

Image #28, page 255, Ina May Gaskin

Image #29, page 256, Ina May Gaskin

Image #30, page 259, U.S. Patent Office, Patent No. 949414, 1910

Image #31, page 260, Janielle Pierucci

Image #32, page 262, Alison Blenkinsop

Image #33, page 263, National Gallery, London

Image #34, page 264, National Gallery, London

Image #35, page 268, Gregory Lowry and Nancy Presly

INDEX

Page numbers of photographs or illustrations appear in *italics*.

B

Baby-Friendly hospitals, 77–79, 253, 276–77, 278
BabyTalk magazine, 261–62
bathing
  boys, foreskin retraction and, 67
  breasts, 65
  breasts, sore, 132, 133
  fathers' help with, 185
  hydrotherapy, 60
  newborns, 65, 66, 70, 82, 207
  oxytocin and, 21
"Bébé Lune," 44
Bedouin culture, 267
benzocaine, 190
beta-endorphin, 23, *24*, 25
bilirubin, 119–20
"biological nurturing," 84–88, *87*, 89
birth, 4, 20. *See also* cesarean birth; labor
  AAP on birth practices, 4
  AAP on first feeding, 4
  attendants and stress, 23, 81
  baby's initial evaluation and, 64–66
  caudal anesthesia, 52
  delayed cord clamping, 62–64
  doula and, 52
  early separation of mother and child, 52
  ecstatic, 60–61
  environment and breastfeeding, 52
  epidural, 52, 58–59, 62, 124
  fetal monitoring, 56
  forceps delivery, 52
  home birth, 82
  hospital birth, 52, 56, 68–79
  Ina May's experience, first child, 52, 70
  information and education about, 55
  magical time just following, 64
  mother's feelings following, 80–81
  1950s–60s, policies developed, 69–70
  oxytocin in mother and child, 20, 22
  pain and, 52
  pain medication, 58–59, 105, 115
  perineal repair, 22–23
  period after birth and bonding, 61–62

placenta (afterbirth) and, 83, 87, 89
positions for labor and delivery, 52
skin-to-skin contact following, 22, 52
stress and, 22–23
uninterrupted time with newborn following, 52
vacuum extraction, 52
birth ball, 60
birth control, 290
  AAP on nursing and, 197
  breastfeeding as, 9, 186–87
  intrauterine devices (IUDs), 197
  pills and decreased milk supply, 196–97
Birth Gazette magazine, 248
Birth journal, 78
bisphenol A (BPA), 166–67, 190
biting, 190–92
  latching problem and, 193
  tips to stop habit, 192–93
  weaning and, 220–21
Blenkinsop, Alison, 263
blogs, 258, 264
blood
  on baby at birth, 81
  drawing, breast milk as analgesic, 8
  infections, 6
  painless bleeding from the breast, 128
  postbirth bleeding, 121, 172, 175
  test for jaundice, 120
bonding, mother-child, 20, 61–62, 65, 69, 71, 81
bone health (mother's), 9, 10, 46–47
bottle-feeding. *See also* milk (artificial)
  avoiding for newborns, 104
  baby's refusal to take a bottle, 176–77
  cost of artificial milk, 10
  environmental impact, 11–12
  fathers and, 8
  health risks of artificial milk, 10–11
  nipples for, 206
  plastics and bottles, 166–67
  refusal of breast and, 117–18
  supplemental feeding for multiples, 206
  tooth decay and, 223
  touch and, 7–8
  WHO on safety of, 5

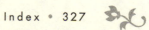

need for, 15, 121–22, 275–79
in Norway, 14, 248–49, 251–57
television proposal, 279

D

Defining Your Own Success (West), 41
dehydration
  of baby, supplemental liquid, 142–43
  diaper count and, 195
  obstructed milk duct and, 131
  signs of, 223
  urine color and, 162
Demerol (meperidine), 23, 59–60, 291
DHA (docosahexaenoic acid), 48–49,
  116, 165
diabetes mellitus, 7
  baby's risk for hypoglycemia and,
    104
  expressed colostrum and, 35
  hand-expressing or pumping breasts
    and, 105
  later lactation and, 105
  milk supply and, 172
diapers
  cloth for newborns, 107
  inspecting to determine amount of
    nutrition ingested, 106–8, 125
  multiples and inspecting, 204
  number of wet per day, 106–8, 125,
    195
  undigested food in, 199
  weight gain and counting, 109, 170
diarrhea, 212–13
  foremilk and, 213
  milk (artificial) and, 6
  when to call the pediatrician, 213
diet and nutrition. *See also* allergies
  breast milk as exclusive, 4, 6, 26,
    197–98, 249
  breast milk for first year, 217
  calcium-rich foods, 46–47
  calories needed for breastfeeding,
    9, 49
  chemical sweeteners, 44
  cravings, 46
  dairy-free diet, 215

fish, advice on eating, 46
foods that affect taste of breast
  milk, 48
how to know you are meeting your
  baby's needs, 106–8
iron-rich foods, 47, 172
natural and organic foods, 44
preparation for nursing, 45–49
protein-rich foods, 44–45
salt, 48
solid foods for baby, 197–99
vegetarians, supplements for, 46
vitamin- and mineral-rich foods, 46
wheat-free diet, 215
dietary and herbal supplements
  alfalfa tablets, 47, 175
  calcium, 46
  DHA, 48–49
  echinacea (for mastitis), 134–36
  herbal, caution, 295–96
  herbal, to increase milk supply,
    174–75
  iron, 47
  nutritional yeast, 46
  taste of breast milk and, 116, 165
  to treat yeast infection, 130
  for vegetarians, 46
Diflucan (fluconazole), 131
digestive tract
  after six months old, 6
  newborns, 6
  solid food introduction and, 6, 198
diuretics, 49, 291
doula, 52, 139, 243
  postpartum, 120, 183, 206

E

ear infection in baby, 195
Easy Expression Bustier, 162
engorgement, 123–24
  epidural and, 124
  mastitis vs., 123–24
  refusal of breast and, 115
  squeeze technique, to reduce, 39, *39*
  tips for reducing symptoms, 124
Environment California, 166–67

Ten Steps to Successful Breastfeeding
protocol, 75–77, 76n
umbilical cord, delayed cutting, 62–64
hospitalization of baby
breastfeeding and, 216–19
breast pumping and, 226
expressed breast milk and, 217, 230
mother's story, 217–19
shared nursing and, 226
support for breastfeeding during, 219
Huggins, Kathleen, 174
hydrotherapy, 60
Hyland's Teething Tablets, 189–90
hypoglycemia, 104
hypothyroidism, 172

I
ibuprofen, 132, 133, 291
iron needs of newborns and mothers, 47

J
Jackson, Janet, 266–67
jaundice, 117, 119–20
colostrum and prevention of, 35
late-preterm baby and, 104
rooming-in and reduced incidence, 71
Jiang Xiaojuan, 21

K
Kane, Susan, 262
Kaneson Comfort Plus pump, 159
kangaroo-care, 66, 73
Kim, Kati, 13–14

L
labor. *See also* doula
breast stimulation and, 35
duration, safe, 57
eating and drinking during, 57
first stage, positions for, 55–56
hospital birth, 57
nonmedical pain remedies, 60–61
pain and position, 55, 56

pain medication, 57–60
positions for, 52, 55–56
shifting poorly positioned baby, 55
lactation (milk production)
beginning of, 27–28
birth-control pills and, 196–97
diabetes or obesity and, 105
drugs to increase supply, 175
emotional upset and suppression,
31–32
employer "lactation program," 153
by grandmothers or women who
haven't been pregnant, 238–47
health conditions that affect, 171–72
herbal supplements to increase, 174–75
higher production, two to six a.m., 29
hormones that affect, 18–25, 51–52
letdown reflex, 28–29
more than enough milk, 113, 177
multiples (twins or more) and, 201
oxytocin and, 28–29, 247
problems, breast surgery and, 39–42
prolactin and, 28
shared nursing and, 226
signs milk has come in, 27–28
slowed, and refusal of breast, 196
spontaneous, 243–47
stimulation of breasts and, 28, 104
stress, effect of, 30–32
too slow weight gain and, 170–71
lactation consultants
after cesarean birth, 202
on circumcision, 68
detection of problems by, 140–41, 174
at hospital, 52
mastitis and, 135
misinformed, 31
for mothers of multiples, 201, 202
sleepy baby problem and, 116
La Leche League (LLL), 38, 276
anti-shared nursing, 230
on breastfeeding after breast surgery, 42
devices available from, 38
educating the medical community on
the value of breast milk, 276
influence on Norway, 252–53
mother education, 237–38

multiples (twins or more) (*cont.*)
  positions for nursing, 205
  prematurity and, 200
  respiratory-distress syndrome, 227–28
  shared nursing and, 227–28
  support for mother and, 200–202, 207
  system to keep track of feeding, 205
  tandem nursing, 210
  umbilical cord clamping and, 63
Muslim societies
  breastfeeding in, *267*, 267–68
  milk siblings, 232
  shared nursing and, 231–32
Mylanta (aluminum hydroxide), 215
myths and lore, 235–47
  by grandmothers or women who
    haven't been pregnant, 238–47
  holes in nipple, for milk, 235–37
  spontaneous lactation, 243–47

N

narcotics and breastfeeding, 59–60, 291
nasal aspirator, 212
Netherlands, maternity-care policy, 122
newborns
  allergies and, 6
  amniotic fluid on, 81
  amount of feeding, 26
  bathing, 65
  behavior change within first days,
    106
  blood sugar level, 26
  blood volume and delayed cutting of
    umbilical cord, 62
  body temperature and
    breastfeeding, 64
  born without medication, 103
  breastfeeding, willingness, 106
  colostrum and, 25–27, 104
  cues for breastfeeding, 85, 91
  diapers and diaper inspection, 106–8
  digestive tract, 6, 25–26
  emotional needs, 108
  first feeding, 4, 70
  first hour of life, 23, 62, 64, 65, 80–81
  first week, needs of, 103–22

growth, 109
how to know you are meeting your
  baby's nutritional needs, 106–8
hunger, lack of in, 105
immunizations, 68
infections, 71
initial evaluation, 64–66, 73
intrinsic reflexes, 84–88, *85*, 115
iron stores in, 47
jaundice, 35
medication in labor and, 58–59, 105
mix-up of, 69
nursing behavior, 193
nuzzling, kissing, licking and, *82*,
  82–83, *83*, 115, 170–71
oxytocin in, 19–20
patience with, 83
placed on mother's abdomen,
  behavior and, 70, 88, 89
poop, first (meconium), 25, 28, 105,
  107
poop of breastfed, 28
position for nursing and, 80, 87, 89
postponement of bathing, testing, eye
  treatments, footprinting, weighing
  and, 66
refusal of breast, 114–18
rooming-in, benefits of, 68–75
separation from mother, hospital
  nursery and, 68–69
skin-to-skin contact following birth
  and, 52, 62, 64, 65, 73, 80, 88, 114
sleep, *72*, 103–4
sling for, 42–43
smell and, 65, 81–82, 116
stored nutrition and survival, 105
sugar water and, 104
umbilical cord, delayed cutting,
  62–64
vernix, 81
weight gain and, 40, 71, 113
weight loss in, 31–32, 40, 105
when to offer your breast, 106
newborns, sick
  AAP on breastfeeding, 4
  colostrum for, 26–27
  ICUs and contact with mother, 66

Newman, Jack, 59
    compression of breast during nursing,
        114
    on drugs to increase milk supply,
        175
    nipple ointment created by, 126, 127
    website, 114
nifedipine, 173, 174
night feedings, 72. *See also* sleeping
    arrangements
    contraceptive benefits of, 187
    importance of, and weight gain, 188
    multiples (twins or more), 207
    number of, 188
    older babies, 195
    weaning and, 223–24
nipplephobia, 266–74
nipples, 162–63
    biting by baby, 190–92
    changes in, when nursing, 18
    checking to prepare for lactation,
        35–38, *36*, *37*, *38*
    colostrum leakage, 34
    cracked or bleeding, 125–27, 133,
        220–21
    exposure to air and sunlight, 35
    holes in, for milk, 235–37
    inverted or retracted, 35–38, *36*, *37*, *38*
    latching and, 97, 98
    milk blister (bleb), 132, 206
    misshapen after nursing and bad latch,
        99, 203
    oil glands and antimicrobial
        environment, 10, 34
    ointments or other applications, 34,
        126–27, 132
    pain during nursing, bad latch and, 99,
        101
    Raynaud's phenomenon and,
        172–74
    sensitivity, paying attention to, 101
    smell and nursing, 81
    soaps, lotions, and, 81
    sore, 125
    sore, bad latch and, 99, 125, 204
    sore, new pregnancy and, 209
    sore, position of baby and, 91

thrush infection, 128–31
    variation of size and shape and
        breastfeeding, 17
nipple shield, 117, *118*, 118–19, 228
No-Cry Sleep Solution, The (Pantley),
    178
Norway
    Baby-Friendly hospitals, 77, 276
    breastfeeding promotion in, 14,
        248–49, 251–57
    percentage of mothers breastfeeding,
        77, 250
    rooming-in, 253
    Vigeland's Sculpture Park, *254*, *255*,
        255–56, *256*
nursing bra, 43
nursing manners for older baby,
    193–95
Nursing Mother's Companion, The
    (Huggins), 174
Nylander, Gro, 77
Nystatin, 130–31

O

obstructed milk duct, 96–97, 131–33
    refusal of breast and, 196
Odent, Michel, 24, 61–62
Of Woman Born (Rich), 181
one- to three-month-old babies, 169–87
    babies' preferences, 176–77
    colic or incessant crying, 177–79
    drugs to increase milk supply, 175
    growth spurt, 169
    health conditions and milk supply,
        171–72
    herbal supplements to increase milk
        supply, 174–75
    mother's lack of sleep and, 180–81
    Raynaud's phenomenon and, 172–74
    slow weight gain, 169–70
    supplemental nursing system, 176
    too much milk for, 177
    wearing your baby, 179
    why baby isn't gaining enough, 170–71
Orgasmic Birth (film), 61
osteoporosis, 9, 46

oxytocin, *19*, 19–23
  "afterpains" and, 9
  analgesic effect, 20
  antihemorrhagic benefits, 9
  breastfeeding and increased, 9
  Chinese earthquake and, 21
  emotions produced by, 19, 21
  healing and, 20, 21
  lactation and, 28–29, 247
  in mammals, 21–22, *22*
  in newborns, 19–20
  in nonpregnant women and men,
    20–21
  released by touch, 21
  skin-to-skin contact and, 20, 22, 71
  stress and, 20, 30–31
  uterus return to pre-pregnant size
    and, 9

P

pacifiers, 171, 215
pain
  acetaminophen for painful nipples, 127
  breast pumping and, 162–63
  cracked/bleeding nipples, 125–27, 133
  ibuprofen for breast pain, 132, 133
  labor position and, 55, 56
  letdown and, 162
  medication, discussion of, 291
  medication during labor, 57–60
  nonmedical remedies for labor, 60–61
  Raynaud's phenomenon and, 172–74
  sore nipples and, 91, 99, 125
Pantley, Elizabeth, 178
perineal repair, 22–23
phthalates, 165–68
PKU screening, 8
placenta (afterbirth), 83, 87, 89, 172
plastics, toxins and, 165–68
  teething rings, what to check, 190
  what to use and what to throw away,
    167–68
Polysporin, 126, 132
positions
  of baby's head, while nursing, *90*,
    90–91, 95, 100

  backache and, 89, 95
  biological nurturing and, 85, 88
  burping, 109, *110*
  carpal tunnel syndrome and, 93, 95
  cradle hold (cuddle hold), 91–93, *92*
  cradle hold (cuddle hold), double,
    205
  cross-cradle hold, 94–95, *96*
  fast milk flow and, 113
  feeding postures, 85, 89
  holding baby, first hour, 80, 87, 89
  to hold or not hold your breast, 97
  for large breasts, 93
  for latching on, 83
  lying position, 89
  multiples, *203*, 203–4, 205
  obstructed milk duct and, 96–97
  for premature babies, 88, 95
  side-lying position, *90*, 90–91
  sitting position, 89–90
  sleeping, for baby, 145–46
  sore nipples and, 91, 95
  underarm and cuddle, two babies,
    205
  underarm hold, 93, *94*, 116, 204
  underarm hold, double, 205
postpartum depression, 122, 181–84
  baby with GERD and, 216
  help and support for, 183
  herbal tea for, 183–84
  risk factors, 182
  rooming-in and reduced incidence, 71
  symptoms, 183
postpartum psychosis, 184
pregnancy. *See also* preparation for
    nursing
  bra advice, 34
  expressing colostrum during, 35
  nursing older baby and, 209–10
premature babies
  AAP on breastfeeding as preferred, 4
  blindness and artificial milk, 6
  breast milk composition and, 5
  expressed colostrum for, 35
  iron supplementation, 47
  kangaroo-care, 66, 73
  late-onset infection, 6

position for nursing and, 88, 95
rooming-in for, 74
touch, need for, 7–8
underarm hold for breastfeeding, 93, *94*
weight gain in, 74, 109
preparation for nursing, 33–50
breast care during pregnancy, 34–35
breastfeeding class, 33
checking nipples, 35–39, *36*, *37*, *38*
dealing with swollen breasts, *39*, 39
dietary needs, 45–49
healthy pregnancy weight, 49–50
lullabies, 44
making your home comfortable, 44
massage or stimulation of breasts, 35
nipple conditioning and, 35
previous breast surgery, 39–42
resistance from family members, dealing with, 33–34
supplies and equipment, 42–44
Prevacid (lansoprazole), 215
Prilosec (omeprazole), 215
problem-solving, first week, 123–43
baby arching away from the breast, 143
baby who needs more fluid, 142–43
cracked or bleeding nipples, 125–28
engorgement, 123–24
mastitis, 133–36
obstructed milk duct, 131–33
painless bleeding from breast, 128
poor tongue habits, 136–37
sore nipples, 125
sucking but not swallowing, 104
tongue-tied baby, 137–42, *138*
yeast or thrush infection, 128–31
progesterone, 24
prolactin, 24–25
beta-endorphin and, 23, 25
contraceptive benefits of, 186–87
drugs that may increase, 175
lactation (milk production) and, 28, 29
skin-to-skin contact and, 71
stress and suppression of, 31
stress reduction and, 25

public breastfeeding
"anti-embarrassment" devices, 258–60, *259*
cover of *BabyTalk* magazine, 261–62
cultural bias against, 250–51
dealing with nipplephobia, 270–74
European countries that support nursing mothers, 250
Facebook banning of photos, 262
harassment of nursing mothers, 250–51, 270–74, 276
legal status in U.S., *272*
Maria Lactans, *263*, 263–66, *264*
nipplephobia, 266–74
Norway and, 249, 253
U.S. cultural repression of, 257–74
U.S. prohibitions on, 249
Walmart and photo, *260*, 260–61
pyloric stenosis, 216

R

Raynaud's phenomenon, 172–74
Reed, Bonnie, 127
refusal of breast, 114–18, 207
arching away from the breast, 143
decreased milk supply, 196–97
engorgement and, 115
expressed milk in cup and, 195
medical reasons, 195–96
mother's story, six months of, 117–18
nipple shield for help with, *118*, 118–19
in older babies, 195–96
slow letdown and, 115
tongue-tie and, 115, 137–42
Reglan (metoclopramide), 175
retinopathy of prematurity, 6
Rich, Adrienne, 181
rickets, 47–48
rooming-in, 68–75
AAP on, 4
availability of, U.S. hospitals, 73
benefits, list of, 71
European hospitals, 74–75, 253
skin-to-skin contact and, 69
U.S., staff attitudes, 75

Sudden Infant Death Syndrome (SIDS)
    breast milk and lowered risk, 7
    outgassing from mattress and, 152
    sleeping position and, 145, 146
    website for more information, 152
supplemental feeding
    AAP on, 4
    avoidance of water, juice, or formula,
        196
    bottle-feeding, 104
    expressed breast milk, 116–17, 196
    lack of, recommended, 26
    multiples (twins or more), 205–7
    previous breast surgery and, 40, 41
    weight loss and, 104
supplemental nursing system (SNS),
        116–17, 176
supplies and equipment
    breast pump, 44
    nursing bra, 43
    sling, 42, 42–43
swaddling, 110–11, 111, 150, 208, 215
    for baby arching away from the
        breast, 143
    skin-to-skin contact vs., 64
    for soothing baby, 178
Sweden, 65, 74–75

T

Tagamet (cimetidine), 215
tandem nursing, 210
teething, 189–90
    common remedies, 189
    homeopathic remedies, 189–90
    over-the-counter remedies, 190
    ring, 190
Ten Steps to Successful Breastfeeding
        protocol, 75–77, 76n, 303–4
thrush, 128–31
    antibiotics and, 117, 129
    Raynaud's phenomenon and, 173
tobacco and nursing, 292
tongue habits, 136–37
tongue-tie, 137–42, 138
    refusal of breast and, 115
tranquilizers, 59, 288–89

travel
    breast pump for, 44
    plane, importance of nursing and, 258
twins. See multiple births

U

umbilical cord
    cord blood banking, 63–64
    delayed clamping of, 62–64
UNICEF
    Code of Marketing of Breast-Milk
        Substitutes, 249
    Ten Steps to Successful Breastfeeding
        protocol, 75–77, 76n
upper respiratory infections/colds, 26
    breast milk and faster recovery, 8
    breast milk and lowered risk, 6
    medication to avoid, 212, 290–91
    nasal congestion, relieving, 212
    nasal congestion and difficulty
        nursing, 211–12
    nasal congestion and refusal of breast,
        195–96
urinary-tract infection, 6, 26
urination
    color of urine and hydration, 162
    wet diapers, daily number, 106–8, 125,
        195
uterine contractions
    afterpains, 9
    breastfeeding and, 89, 209
    oxytocin and, 9

V

vacuum extraction, 52
vaporizer, cool-mist, 195–96, 212
vernix, 81
videos on nursing, 33
Vigeland, Gustav, 254, 255, 255–57, 256
vitamin B12, 46
vitamin D, 47–48
vomiting, 216
    food reactions and, 48
    GERD and, 213
    projectile, 216

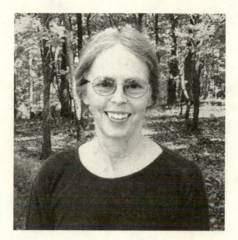

INA MAY GASKIN, certified professional midwife, has been a midwife for more than thirty-five years at The Farm Midwifery Center at The Farm, in Summertown, Tennessee. Nearly 100 percent of the women who have given birth and lived in the Farm community have been able to exclusively breastfeed their babies. Ina May is past president of the Midwives' Alliance of North America. She lectures internationally, writes for national publications, and has been interviewed by a range of media on birth and breastfeeding.